Trauma and the Anaesthetist

Trauma and the Anaesthetist

J.C. STODDART

MD, FFARCS
Consultant Anaesthetist and Consultant in Charge
Intensive Therapy Unit
Royal Victoria Infirmary
Newcastle upon Tyne

WITH CONTRIBUTIONS BY

N.E.F. CARTLIDGE

MBBS, FRCP
Consultant Neurologist and Senior Lecturer in Neurology
Royal Victoria Infirmary
Newcastle upon Tyne

AND

L.J. DUNKIN

MBBCh, FFARCS
Consultant Anaesthetist
The General Hospital
Newcastle upon Tyne

Baillière Tindall

LONDON PHILADELPHIA TORONTO MEXICO CITY
RIO DE JANEIRO SYDNEY TOKYO HONG KONG

Baillière Tindall 1 St Anne's Road
Eastbourne, East Sussex BN21 3UN, England

West Washington Square
Philadelphia, PA 19105, USA

1 Goldthorne Avenue
Toronto, Ontario M8Z 5T9, Canada

Apartado 26370—Cedro 512
Mexico 4, D.F., Mexico

Rua Evaristo da Veiga, 55–20° andar
Rio de Janeiro—RJ, Brazil

ABP Australia Ltd, 44 Waterloo Road
North Ryde, NSW 2064, Australia

Ichibancho Central Building, 22-1 Ichibancho
Chiyoda-ku, Tokyo 102, Japan

10/FL, Inter-Continental Plaza, 94 Granville Road
Tsim Sha Tsui East, Kowloon, Hong Kong

First published 1984

Typeset and printed in Great Britain at The Alden Press, Oxford
Bound by Mackays of Chatham

British Library Cataloguing in Publication Data

Stoddart, J.C.
  Trauma and the anaesthetist.
  1. Anaesthesia   2. Traumatism
  I. Title   II. Cartlidge, N.E.F.
  III. Dunkin, L.J.
  617'.21   RD87

ISBN 0 7020 1041 3

Contents

Preface

Although the anaesthetist's principal responsibility is for the patient in the operating room, recently his activities have broadened to include the intensive therapy unit and the pain clinic. In many hospitals he has also become involved in administrative and clinical duties in the casualty department and with casualty evacuation and handling. These developments have followed naturally from his operating room duties.

Originally, the anaesthetist was expected to provide safe anaesthesia for patients who were undergoing relatively undemanding surgical procedures, but the ambitions of the surgeon grew in parallel with the skills of the anaesthetist and in particular with his knowledge of respiratory support and cardiocirculatory resuscitation. As a direct consequence of these developments he was expected to make decisions as to the patient's fitness to undergo anaesthesia and surgery and to recommend the appropriate pre-anaesthetic preparation. The next stage arose out of his responsibility for the patient's post-operative state; in the first instance this was restricted to a decision as to whether or not the patient was fit to leave the protected environment of the operating room. This led to the provision of recovery room facilities, and gradually the anaesthetist's participation grew so that his election to responsibility for patients in the intensive therapy unit was both inevitable and logical.

In this book, the anaesthetist's contribution to the care of the traumatized patient is discussed. In this context, trauma is taken to mean injuries which result from external violence, which include, in addition to the obvious causes, burns, drowning, exposure and hypothermia.

The anaesthetist is involved with the traumatized patient at all stages. In the first place, he may be called to the casualty department to assist with the resuscitation of the critically ill patient who has been injured in some way which threatens his survival. He may also be concerned with the organization of first-aid services in which his involvement ranges from teaching members of the rescue services to his personal inclusion in the major accident team.

In some parts of Europe, and particularly in France, the accident and emergency department of a hospital is under the administrative and clinical charge of an anaesthetist or of a specialist whose basic postgraduate training is in anaesthesia. With the current expansion of accident and emergency services, this is increasingly the case in the United Kingdom. The handling and transportation of patients in specialized vehicles, which range from unmodified ambulances to helicopters and fixed wing aircraft, may also be his responsibility to a greater or lesser extent. In the United Kingdom, the obvious example of this is the Royal Air Force 'Casevac' system, which is largely the anaesthetist's province.

In the operating room the anaesthetist has to provide anaesthesia for patients who have sustained a wide variety of injuries while they undergo what may be very extensive and traumatic surgery. The pre-operative assessment of these patients is more than usually important because, in addition to the external injuries, he must be able to recognize the development of signs of unsuspected injury whilst the patient is anaesthetized. Examples of these include intra-abdominal bleeding and the development of a tension pneumo-thorax or of the signs of an extradural haemorrhage whilst the patient may be undergoing a relatively mundane orthopaedic or facio-maxillary procedure.

Penetrating wounds and injuries caused by high explosives are mentioned briefly in the relevant chapters, although their management does not differ qualitatively from that of injuries which have a less dramatic cause.

This book is intended to provide a practical guide to the management of the traumatized patient and it is hoped that anaesthetists at all stages in their careers will find it to be of value. It should also be of use to casualty officers and those who are concerned with the organization of emergency rescue services.

In some of the succeeding chapters a variety of technical manoeuvres is described. Examples of these include trans-tracheal insufflation, the use of the fibre-optic bronchoscope for difficult intubation, and the place of thoracic epidural analgesia in the treatment of chest injuries. It is not supposed that trainees will be able to learn how to perform these techniques from a book of this type. However, the fact that such methods have been used successfully on many occasions should encourage them to practise them under supervision whenever the opportunity arises.

J. C. Stoddart

Acknowledgements

It is a pleasure to acknowledge the contributions made to this book by Dr N.E.F. Cartlidge and Dr L.J.Dunkin. Dr Cartlidge is a Consultant Neurologist and Senior Lecturer in Neurology in the University of Newcastle upon Tyne and he has made a special study of coma and its prognosis. Dr Dunkin is a Consultant Anaesthetist who is attached to the Regional Burns Unit at Newcastle General Hospital and he has a comprehensive knowledge of the problems presented by the patient with severe burn injuries. No book on trauma would be complete without sections devoted to these subjects.

The manuscript was patiently prepared by my secretary, Mrs E.F. Blacklock, and most of the illustrations were produced by the staff of the Audio-Visual Aids Centre, University of Newcastle upon Tyne; for their skill I am very grateful.

J.C.S.

1

Priorities in the Care of
the Injured Patient

All medical care is based upon the assessment of priorities. Whether the attendant is faced with a single casualty or a large number, the initial objective is to decide how to deal most effectively with the clinical problem. This process is called triage (sorting) and it is at its most elementary when many casualties have to be dealt with, when it may be concerned only with the immediate treatment of life-threatening conditions. However, it must be more detailed and comprehensive if only one patient is involved.

Individual triage

The medical attendant who is presented with a traumatized patient must ask himself the following questions:
1 Which injury is most life-threatening and requires *immediate* treatment?
2 Which injury can be left until a later *time* but should be treated urgently?
3 Which injury can safely be left until a later *date* and be treated electively?

The assessment of priorities must be performed as soon as possible by the most senior person present, but it is a continuous process which should be repeated at frequent short intervals so that any new development can be recognized. Injuries which involve the respiratory tract are more immediately life-threatening than are other types of injury, with the possible exception of major arterial or venous bleeding. It is commonly stated that a patient who is bleeding is probably breathing: the corollary to this is that a patient who is bleeding still has blood circulating. It is usually not difficult to determine the immediate priority and in any case the insertion of an artificial airway (oral airway; nasopharyngeal airway; endotracheal tube) should take only a moment. Whoever first sees the patient must be prepared to perform first aid, whether this is to support the airway, perform endotracheal intubation, apply controlled ventilation or arrest external bleeding. The use of pressure dressings, artery clips or tourniquets should be within the scope of every medical or paramedical attendant. The emergency treatment of chest injuries is described in Chapter 4 but may include the application of an occlusive dressing over a penetrating or sucking wound or the insertion of a chest drainage tube.

Record-keeping

At many points in this book the importance of good record-keeping will be emphasized. In the most dire emergency the medical attendant can glance at his watch and make a mental note of the time of certain vital events, even if he has to document them a little later. Ideally he would record them at the time and mini-tape recorders may be used for this purpose in the field. In hospital the major disaster plan, which is referred to later, must include the provision of secretarial staff to accompany the clinician and note his observations.

As much information as possible should be obtained from the patient since, in addition to its relevance to his present state, it may be of medicolegal importance. Unfortunately, all too often observations which have both diagnostic and prognostic significance are noted either casually and illegibly or not at all. All written notes must be legible, dated, timed and signed.

INITIAL OBSERVATIONS

The minimum number of observations which must be recorded are:

1 The patient's full name, age and sex. Sometimes these data are not immediately obtainable, but other identifying marks must be recorded. An essential part of the equipment of the major accident team is a supply of tie-on labels which should be attached to patients and used for identification and to record the dose, route and time of drugs given (which *must* include any narcotic drugs).

2 The time and place of the first contact with the patient.

3 His state of consciousness.

4 His ability to maintain a clear airway and breathe adequately.

5 His cardiocirculatory state, together with evidence of blood loss.

6 His ability (or inability) to move all four limbs on request or in response to stimulation.

7 The position (central/deviated/divergent) size, equality and reactivity of his pupils.

8 The list of the investigations which have been requested.

Patients who have been involved in accidents of any kind are frequently distressed, excited or in severe pain. However, it is essential not to obscure important physical signs by giving analgesic or sedative drugs before as much information as possible has been obtained from the patient. This particularly relates to evidence of occult injury involving the head, thoracic cage and abdomen. As soon as the medical attendant is reasonably confident that he is not in danger of missing such an injury the patient can be given the appropriate sedative or analgesic drug. The choice is wide and the topic is discussed later in this chapter.

As soon as possible the patient should be undressed completely and examined from head to toe, particular attention being paid to the back and perineum, regions which are commonly examined cursorily or not at all. The author has vivid memories of an unconscious road traffic accident victim who had filled his trouser legs and both of his rubber boots with his blood before it was realized he was exsanguinating from a groin wound.

The assessment of respiratory function

Estimation of the adequacy of respiration is most difficult, and many medical attendants seem to consider that if a patient is breathing at all he is breathing adequately. The observer must make note of the patency of the airway, which includes evidence of localized bleeding, swelling or the presence of foreign material. The rate and rhythm of respiration must also be noted, since the latter may give early evidence of intracranial damage. The depth of respiration is most difficult to assess and even experienced observers are commonly misled.

Skin colour

Patients who have been involved in accidents or fires are usually very dirty and this makes the assessment of skin colour very difficult or impossible. It is usually stated that the colour of the tongue is a useful guide to the patient's state of oxygenation, but this may be unreliable because of blood loss, dryness, bleeding in the mouth or pharynx, or furring of the tongue. If there is any suspicion as to the adequacy of ventilation and oxygenation, blood gas measurement is the only really reliable indicator and should be carried out as soon as the patient reaches hospital. This is one of the routine laboratory investigations which all such patients should undergo. Others are listed later in this chapter.

Respiratory support

If the assessment of respiratory adequacy is being undertaken at the site of the incident no laboratory tests can be performed, and if there is any doubt about the state of the respiratory system, the airway and respiratory activity must be supported. Every patient who is unconscious or stuporose must be assumed to be in danger of asphyxia or of ventilatory failure. There should be no need to emphasize the importance of nursing such a patient on his side, preferably $10°$ head down. If the full physical examination has not yet been completed the patient's airway may need to be supported while he is lying on his back.

If the stuporose patient will tolerate an anaesthetic airway he needs one. This may suggest that laryngoscopy, followed by endotracheal intubation, is required. This subject is discussed more fully in Chapter 3. An efficient suction device is an absolutely essential part of the emergency equipment and modern portable foot-operated suckers are almost as efficient as are those driven by piped gases or electricity. Portable vacuum suckers are of limited value since they soon become exhausted.

Less obvious respiratory injuries

External injuries may be obvious, but less gross changes such as limited abdominal movement, which may suggest internal injuries, or minor degrees of paradoxical ventilation, require more careful observation in a good light. The examination should commence with the attendant standing at the foot of the couch and looking upwards along the length of the patient's body. From this position, obstructed, exaggerated or other abnormal respiratory movements can be easily recognized. These include the use of the accessory muscles of respiration and uneven chest movements.

Surgical emphysema may be obvious, but it may not be recognized until the medical attendant either palpates the patient's chest or applies his stethoscope to it, when the typical crackling noises are heard. This usually means that the patient has a pneumothorax, but injury to other intrathoracic structures—such as to the trachea or bronchus or to the oesophagus—may occasionally be responsible. Not infrequently no source of surgical emphysema is found, and it has to be assumed that the air has tracked from inside the damaged lung, through adherent pleura, into the subcutaneous tissues.

The cardiocirculatory system

A patient who has suffered a large volume blood loss will show signs of cardiocirculatory disturbance. These are discussed in Chapter 2, but at the initial examination, which may need to be performed at the same time as treatment is being instituted, certain vital points must be noted. These include the external injuries, but as well as recording the pulse rate and rhythm and blood pressure, the examiner must palpate all major pulses and note their presence or absence; these include the carotid, brachial, radial, femoral, popliteal and dorsalis pedis pulses on both sides of the body. Observation of skin temperature and perfusion are unreliable if the patient is cold or dirty, but if an obvious discrepancy between two limbs is recognized this must be noted.

Superficial neurological examination

As part of the initial examination, the attendant should ask the patient to move his arms, hands, legs and feet and to indicate that he has proprioceptive, pain and touch sensation. This may be very difficult if the patient has limb injuries, particularly if these have been splinted, bandaged, or covered in plaster of paris and if any doubt exists a neurologist's opinion should be obtained as soon as possible (Chapter 8).

Covert injuries

A patient who has suffered pelvic or intra-abdominal injuries may be shocked as a result of occult blood loss, but in addition he may be anuric or be unable to pass urine. No matter how anxious the medical attendant may be to measure and record the patient's urinary output, urethral or bladder neck injuries must be excluded before a urinary catheter is inserted (Chapter 10).

The patient's posture may be a guide to diagnosis even when his level of consciousness is impaired. His hands may cover or point to a painful area; if one or both lower limbs are held in a position of external rotation or flexion this should make the attendant think of femoral neck or shaft injury and try to confirm or exclude these before moving the patient. Photophobia suggests either ocular or cerebral damage; muscular rigidity usually protects a painful area.

Clothing marks (those in which the pattern of the garment can be seen) on the chest or abdomen imply that the impact has been very violent, and should make the attendant consider the likelihood of internal injuries (page 170).

THE INJURY SEVERITY SCORE

Although the initial treatment of the traumatized patient is based upon the assessment of priorities, it is important if possible to quantify the extent of the injury or injuries, for three reasons. In the first instance, this allows the patient's medical attendant to assess the probable outcome and plan the course of treatment more accurately; in the second place, classification permits the effects of different methods of treatment to be compared; finally, it enables the medical attendant to give a more accurate prognosis to the patient or his next of kin.

The Maryland Scoring System

The scoring system which originated from the Maryland Institute for Emergency Medicine is probably the best known. It is based upon the prospective analysis of more than 2000 trauma victims in which numerical values were given to injuries to different parts of the body (1 to 5 in order of severity). Similar systems have been described, but they were found to be of limited value because they failed to quantify the additive effects of injuries affecting more than one part of the body. For example, it became apparent that a patient who had two grade 4 injuries did not necessarily have the same prognosis as a patient with one grade 5 and one grade 3 injury.

The Maryland workers recognized that the effects of injuries were related in a quadratic fashion. The system is based upon the classification of injuries to the head and neck, thorax, abdomen, pelvis and extremities into one of five categories:

Grade 1—minor.
Grade 2—moderate.
Grade 3—severe, but not life-threatening.
Grade 4—severe, life-threatening, survival probable.
Grade 5—critical, survival uncertain.

Only the three most severely injured regions are included in the assessment. The individual totals are then squared and added together—for example:

Multiple rib fractures with respiratory impairment:	$4 \times 4 = 16$
Compound fracture of temporal bone with brain exposure:	$4 \times 4 = 16$
Ruptured spleen and lacerated liver:	$3 \times 3 = 9$

Total 41

The additional effect of age has also been estimated (Figure 1). This figure, which shows the overall survival rates for different scores and age groups, also demonstrates that the most pronounced effect of ageing is noted in the lower injury score ranges.

This type of classification is widely used and is particularly valuable in

MORTALITY BY INJURY SEVERITY SCORE FOR THREE AGE GROUPS.
DOA's EXCLUDED FROM CALCULATIONS.
DOTTED LINES CONNECT POINTS BASED UPON LESS THAN 10 PERSONS.

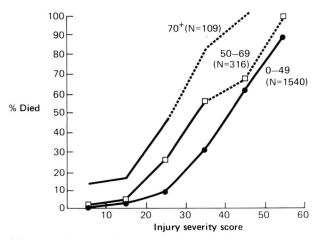

Figure 1. The 'injury severity score': effects of age. The mortality rate for patients with scores greater than 50 is very high. However, no scoring system should be allowed to influence the initial resuscitative efforts.

epidemiological studies of the effects of multiple injuries. However, its predictive value for all but the most destructive injuries is less than 95%, and the medical attendant must not allow classification to influence the determination with which he pursues resuscitative measures.

Patient handling

Many injuries are exacerbated by thoughtless handling, and the possibility of the most dangerous ones should be excluded—if necessary by radiography—before the patient is moved. The obvious examples of this type of injury include cervical and lumbar spine fractures which may cause permanent neurological damage if the patient is moved thoughtlessly. Pelvic and femoral shaft fractures always cause extensive blood loss which is aggravated by excessive movement.

All medical and paramedical staff should understand these points. When moving patients, either at the accident site or in hospital, only trained personnel should be involved. Ideally, five people should be available to move each injured patient so that he can be lifted 'in one piece'. One attendant must concentrate all his attention on the patient's head and neck; the patient's head should rest between this attendant's forearms while his hands support the shoulders. If a comprehensive examination has excluded injuries of the kind described above, patient handling may be simplified but should always be considerate.

Several types of specialized stretcher are available for extricating and moving traumatized patients from the site of the incident. They are designed for portability and to take up as little space as possible, while at the same time enveloping the patient in a semi-rigid cocoon. Any doctor who is potentially part of a major accident team should familiarize himself with these and other pieces of equipment which he may have to use.

Other details of patient handling, together with transport and monitoring in transit, are considered later in this book (Chapter 11).

PLANNING FOR MAJOR DISASTERS

A major accident is usually defined as one from which a minimum of 25 survivors is expected. This is a rather arbitrary classification, since a small hospital may be overwhelmed by the arrival of less than half this number of patients. Nevertheless most teaching hospitals and district general hospitals use this definition, and have adopted a policy to deal with such an eventuality.

Aims and objectives

In detail, the major accident policy is a local affair, designed to fulfil projected local needs. The hospital which serves an airport or railway terminal will plan for a different type of emergency from one which sits beside a motorway, daily expecting the results of a football coach accident, or which is situated beside an industrial complex. In some 'front line' cities the victims of civil strife or of terrorist activities must also be considered. However, the aims of every major accident plan are identical, namely:
1 To provide on-site first aid.
2 To organize the safe transportation of casualties.
3 To prepare efficient hospital reception services.

Although every doctor hopes that he will never be involved in a major disaster, at the same time he believes implicitly that he will know what to do in the unlikely event. Nevertheless, prior planning for such an eventuality is essential. Hospitals which are isolated must be prepared to act independently, but it is usual for two adjacent city hospitals to share the responsibility for the actions which are required. The casualty consultants of the relevant hospitals must ensure that the plans are kept up to date and their contents distributed to all personnel who may be involved. Mock disaster exercises should be planned and taken very seriously. It is important for the doctor and nurse to recognize that in this type of situation they play a secondary role and are at the disposal of the professionals, i.e., the police, fire brigade and ambulance services.

In the event of a major disaster one of the paired hospitals will be designated the first-line hospital and the other the supporting hospital. The choice of the first-line hospital depends upon the location of the emergency. The decision that a major disaster has occurred is made by either the Senior Police Officer or the Senior Ambulance Officer at the site of the incident, who informs the hospital switchboard.

Outline plan

The details of the arrangements made thereafter are determined in advance by the local planning team, and a document setting out these arrangements should be published within the paired hospitals. The switchboard is the focal point of the emergency and all the telephonists must know the actions which they have to take.

1   The telephone switchboard of the first-line hospital must have a list of the personnel to be informed.

2   Key members of the emergency team must keep a list of telephone numbers of secondary personnel who may need to be informed should circumstances require it.

3   Preliminary plans must have been made for clearing reception areas and preparing for surgical operations and patient admission. These are put into effect.

4   The police will provide transport to take a Site Medical Officer from the first-line hospital to the incident site. He is usually the senior surgical registrar on duty.

5   The duty of the Site Medical Officer is to assess the severity of the incident. He will establish and maintain contact with his home base by radio. The radio link is provided by the police. If he decides it is necessary, he will ask for one or more mobile medical teams to be despatched to the site. He will also keep the Major Disaster Officer informed of the flow of casualties and their condition, and particularly of any gravely injured patient who is on his way to hospital.

6   The first Mobile Medical Team is provided by the supporting hospital. It consists of an anaesthetist (usually a senior registrar), a house officer and two nurses. At the discretion of the Site Medical Officer additional mobile medical teams can be sent. Transport is provided by the police or ambulance services.

7   The hospital administration must be prepared to provide additional personnel to aid patient movement, handle enquiries from relatives and others, and be responsible for record-keeping, including the registration of deaths. Additional hospital telephone numbers may be required and a press-room established. The hospital chaplain must be informed of the situation.

8   Large numbers of walking wounded and uninjured individuals may be brought to the Casualty Department of the first-line hospital. These will create chaos unless they are firmly and efficiently handled. A department which can easily be emptied, such as the physiotherapy gymnasium, should be set aside for this purpose. (On one occasion 103 patients were brought to the author's hospital following the derailment of an express train. Only five patients required admission.)

9   The co-ordination of these services is the responsibility of the Major Disaster Officer. He (or his deputy) is the consultant in charge of the accident and emergency department of the first-line hospital. He must make a point of maintaining contact with his colleagues at the supporting hospital.

Clinical activities

The responsibilities of the Major Disaster Officer and his staff in the hospital were outlined at the beginning of this chapter. These are triage, resuscitation and the correct disposal of the injured. The Site Medical Officer and the Mobile Medical Team have a relatively restricted field of clinical activity, viz: the assessment and treatment of life-threatening emergencies affecting the airway, breathing, and circulation. Rarely, aid may be required to facilitate the extrication of a trapped victim. This may include the amputation of a badly damaged limb which is preventing his release from a dangerous environment.

It should be emphasized at this point that the release and extrication of patients is the responsibility of the rescue services who are trained for these tasks. Enthusiastic but inept personnel merely get in the way.

Resuscitation

Medical personnel give physical assistance only at the request of the rescue team leader. However, resuscitation procedures may be needed at the accident site before the patient is moved. These include the administration of oxygen, blood volume expanders and analgesics. Mouth-to-mouth or bag-and-mask ventilation, or endotracheal intubation, may be required. It may be necessary to arrest major bleeding or to apply a pack to a sucking chest wound before the patient is moved. Exceptionally, a tension pneumothorax may need to be released, although this condition is hard to recognize and underwater seal drainage is very difficult to maintain in the field. If a chest drain has to be inserted, dry drainage with the aid of a Heimlich valve or similar device is more satisfactory (Figure 2).

The indications for most types of emergency surgery depend to some extent on the distance the patient has to be transported. A balance must be struck between the immediate needs of the patient and the realization that most procedures can safely be delayed. Unless very specialized transport is

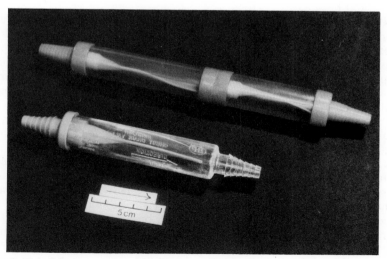

Figure 2. Heimlich-type one-way valve for chest drainage (top, Viggon; bottom, Bard Parker).

used, only a minimum of procedures can be performed in transit. The airway must be guaranteed and any intravenous infusion fastened securely. The ambulance must have an adequate supply of the appropriate intravenous fluids to last out the journey, which may take much longer than is anticipated. If many critically ill patients have to be transported, the Site Medical Officer must request further assistance so that each patient can be accompanied by a competent anaesthetist. These and other problems presented by transportation are discussed in Chapter 11.

Miscellaneous problems

The organization of a major disaster team must take account of practical problems such as the clothing the team should wear, the provision of emergency lighting, and the storage, handling and responsibility for dangerous drugs and similar items which have legal restrictions to their use or limited shelf-life.

Experience suggests that clothing should be waterproof, brightly coloured and labelled in extremely large letters with the wearer's function (i.e., Nurse, Doctor, etc.). Wellington boots, portable back-packs and heavy duty torches are an essential part of any team's equipment. Area lighting is provided by the rescue services.

The choice of the drugs and equipment to be taken to the accident site is a matter for the team to decide in advance. However, many of the items which may be used are mentioned in this and subsequent chapters.

The employing authority must insure all members of the team in case of accidents or death occurring in transit or at the accident site.

ANAESTHESIA AND ANALGESIA FOR EXTRICATION AND TRANSPORTATION

The drugs which are used in an emergency should be kept to a minimum. This is particularly the case with analgesic and anaesthetic agents which may have undesirable side-effects upon the injured patient. The administration of anaesthesia in all but the most ideal circumstances is potentially hazardous. Anyone who has been forced to anaesthetize patients at accident sites or in the field of military operations agrees that it is best avoided, but if essential it should be as uncomplicated as possible.

The use of ketamine

Various techniques have been used, but at present the agent of choice is ketamine combined with oxygen by face-mask from a portable system. Ketamine has several advantages. In the first place, in sub-anaesthetic doses it is an effective analgesic and amnesic with minimal side-effects. For this purpose the dose range should be from 0.5–1 mg/kg body weight (40–80 mg ketamine for an adult). This will permit injured patients to be moved without dangerous side-effects or memorable distress. The emphasis on memory is important, because although patients who must be moved may show signs of discomfort at the time, if they have been given ketamine in this dosage range they appear to have no recollection of the event 30 minutes later.

Ketamine has the additional advantage of being effective when given by either intramuscular or intravenous routes, although when given intramuscularly the initial dose should be at the upper end of the scale recommended above. It is frequently impossible to give intravenous injections (or erect intravenous infusions) at the accident site until the patient has been moved to a controllable location, such as an ambulance or other shelter nearby. The occasional dysphoric effects of ketamine may be unfortunate, but these are outweighed by its other good qualities. These include the fact that it rarely causes respiratory depression.

If an intravenous infusion or access point is available and full anaesthesia is required, ketamine should be given intravenously in an initial dose of 1.5–2.0 mg/kg body weight. Before giving ketamine it is essential to know if the patient has already received a narcotic analgesic such as morphine or pethidine. This information should have been recorded on the label attached to the patient. Traumatized patients react unpredictably to analgesic and narcotic drugs, and the combination of opiates and ketamine often causes respiratory depression which can be lethal.

Route of administration

Where possible all potent drugs should be given intravenously so that their effects can be assessed quickly. The choice of analgesic drugs for the traumatized patient is almost limitless, but unless ketamine is used as described above most experienced clinicians rely upon morphine, papaveretum or pethidine, given intravenously in incremental doses, because they are such predictable agents within the limits of the circumstances in which they are used.

Opiate narcotics should only be given by intramuscular injection as a last resort since their absorption may be delayed as a result of hypothermia or vasoconstriction. Subcutaneous injections must never be given.

Other agents which have been used or recommended for emergency anaesthesia at the accident site include barbiturates, etomidate or entonox. The undesirable effects of the barbiturates are self-evident and they should never be used in the field. Etomidate may have a place for the induction of anaesthesia for the shocked patient in a protected environment such as a casualty department or operating room but it cannot be given intramuscularly, it has no analgesic properties and may give rise to undesirable muscle movements. It is said to cause few cardiocirculatory effects but this cannot be guaranteed; its longer term use may cause suprarenal depression. Entonox is often recommended and many ambulances carry it routinely. It undoubtedly has a place in the treatment of mild to moderately severe pain, provided that the patient can learn to handle the equipment, which is often not possible; a more important practical problem may be getting the apparatus to the trapped patient. For the patient in severe pain its effects are marginal, but it does guarantee effective oxygenation.

Neuromuscular blocking agents

The need for the use of relaxants in the field should be exceptional, but ketamine together with atracurium or pancuronium, followed by endotracheal intubation, offers the safest combination. Ventilation may be controlled with an Ambu bag or similar device until more formal means are available.

In hospital, the choice of anaesthetic technique for the traumatized patient is governed by standard anaesthetic practice. Some specific problems may arise. These are discussed in the relevant chapters which follow.

References

Baker, S.P., O'Neill, B., Haddon, W. & Long, W.B. (1974) The injury severity score: a method for describing patients with multiple injuries and evaluating emergency care. *Journal of Trauma*, **14**(3), 187–196.

Bond, A.C. & Davies, C.K. (1974) Ketamine and pancuronium for the shocked patient. *Anaesthesia*, **29**, 59–62.

Chasapalius, G., Kakis, N., Sakkalis, C. & Dohol, D. (1973) Use of ketamine and pancuronium for anesthesia for patient in haemorrhagic shock. *Anesthesia and Analgesia; Current Researches*, **52**(2), 282–287.

Finch, P. & Nancekievill, D. (1975) The role of hospital mobile medical teams at a major accident. *British Journal of Hospital Medicine*, **5**, 601–610.

Folsam, F. (1975) *Casualty Handling Techniques*. 150 pp. Philadelphia and Toronto: J.B. Lippincott.

Hindle, J.F. (1978) The management of multiple injuries. *British Journal of Hospital Medicine*, **3**, 219–223.

Macmahon, A.C. (1977) Medical management of the trapped patient. *South African Medical Journal*, **52**, 683–685.

Richardson, J.W. (1975) *Disaster Planning*. 121 pp. Bristol: Wright.

Snook, R. (1974) *Medical Aid at Accidents*. 130 pp. London: Update Publications.

2

Shock: Acute Cardiocirculatory Failure

Shock is a complex phenomenon, and in a book of this type only a summary of present ideas as to its causes and treatment can be given. Although many definitions have been attempted, it is best described by its effect, namely, failure of the cardiocirculatory system to satisfy the metabolic needs of organs and tissues. These needs include: (1) the delivery of oxygen, nutrients and other substances, and (2) the removal of organic and inorganic waste products. The results of failure are tissue starvation and auto-intoxication.

The causes of shock are usually separated into three main groups. Haemorrhagic shock is caused by the sudden loss of a major percentage (more than 25%) of the circulating blood volume. Cardiogenic shock follows infarction of a large mass of left ventricular muscle. Septicaemic shock is more complex; it results either from an overwhelming infection or from failure of the body's defences to cope with a less obvious microbial invasion. Patients with shock due to haemorrhage or myocardial infarction always have a reduced cardiac output initially, whereas patients with shock due to sepsis have a normal or raised cardiac output until the terminal phase. Cardiogenic shock is not considered further in this book. Septicaemic shock will be discussed in some detail since it may complicate trauma and its treatment.

HAEMORRHAGIC SHOCK

Haemorrhagic shock has two phases, the first of which is caused by the activation of the baroreceptor mechanism following a sudden fall of the cardiac output. This can be readily reversed if the cause is recognized and treated quickly and efficiently, but if not, the patient may enter the second phase which is characterized by organ and tissue damage and which may have serious long-term consequences.

The baroreceptor system (Figure 3) is designed to cope with demands for short-term changes in the cardiac output and blood pressure such as those which may follow a change in posture from the horizontal to the vertical position or running from a standing start. Under these circumstances it works well, but it is not intended to cope with a sustained demand. The components of the system are: (1) the medullary vasomotor centre (VMC); (2) baroreceptors in the aortic arch, carotid sinus, great veins and atria; and (3) the hypothalamus and autonomic nervous system. Other parts are played by the renal juxtaglomerular apparatus, the suprarenal glands, the hypothalamus

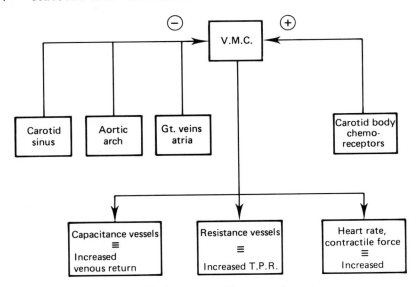

Figure 3. The baroreceptor/chemoreceptor system.

and pituitary glands. The carotid body chemoreceptors may also be involved since they are activated by hypoxia, hypercapnia and acidaemia.

Under resting conditions the vasomotor centre is in a state of tonic inhibition. If, for any reason, the cardiac output falls, the number of inhibitory impulses which originate in the baroreceptors is reduced and the vasomotor centre releases excitatory stimuli through the sympathetic nervous system. These are responsible for the clinical features of shock which include:

1 Pallor
2 Cold moist skin
3 Tachycardia
4 Increased force of cardiac contraction
5 Rise in total peripheral resistance (TPR)
6 Contraction of capacitance vessels
7 Selective diversion of blood flow
8 Oliguria

The resistance vessels are the small arteries and arterioles. The capacitance vessels are the large arteries and veins. Normally, two-thirds of the blood volume is contained within the capacitance system. Its contraction temporarily increases the venous return and this is augmented by more complete ventricular emptying. Selective vasoconstriction causes blood to be diverted from the splanchnic vessels and the kidneys to areas which are more immediately vital, including the heart, brain and voluntary muscles. As a result of renal vasoconstriction, together with the effects of the secretion of antidiuretic hormone, aldosterone and cortisol, the patient becomes oliguric.

In spite of appreciable blood loss these mechanisms allow the cardiac output to be maintained or even increased temporarily. The blood pressure may fall only minimally but at the cost of a marked reduction in peripheral and splanchnic perfusion. This relationship is demonstrated by the equation:

$$BP = \dot{Q} \times TPR$$

Where BP = the systemic blood pressure, $\dot{Q}$ = the cardiac output (l/min), and TPR = the total peripheral resistance.

Cortisol secretion is increased because of hypothalamic stimulation, and that of aldosterone when perfusion of the intrathoracic baroreceptors falls. ADH (vasopressin) is secreted in response to a rise in serum osmolality (provided this is not caused by an increased concentration of freely diffusible substances, such as urea). Renal perfusion falls as a consequence of the fall in systemic blood pressure and vasoconstriction; renin is released from the juxtaglomerular apparatus, and the precursor angiotensin I is converted to angiotensin II. This is a powerful vasoconstrictor which also stimulates aldosterone secretion.

Together, these factors cause sodium and water retention so as to maintain the circulating blood volume; as a result the patient passes a small volume of concentrated urine.

The Starling diagram

Figure 4 (the Starling diagram) is a simplified representation of the balance between the intravascular (hydrostatic) pressure and the plasma oncotic pressure. Under normal circumstances the excess hydrostatic pressure at the arteriolar end of the capillary forces fluid outwards; at the venular end, the plasma oncotic pressure draws it back into the circulation. When the systemic blood pressure falls, or when local factors cause the pre-capillary sphincter to close, the hydrostatic pressure falls below the oncotic pressure and fluid is drawn into the circulation throughout the length of the capillary. This increases the blood volume, but at the same time it limits the transport of nutrients to the tissues. The diagram emphasizes the importance of the oncotic pressure, most of which is generated by the serum albumin.

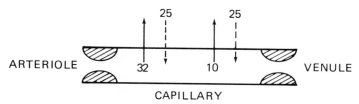

Figure 4. The Starling diagram. The figures represent the hydrostatic (———►) and oncotic (– – ►) pressures involved in water and solute exchange. The shaded areas show the positions of the functional sphincters.

The vascular unit

The distribution of blood to the tissues and organs is not a haphazard arrangement but is through vascular units. Figure 5 represents an idealized

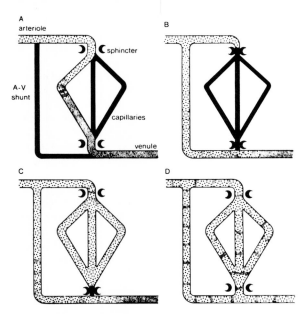

Figure 5. The four stages of the vasoconstrictor response to a sudden fall in cardiac output. For a full description see text.

vascular unit at various stages after activation of the vasomotor centre. Each unit consists of an arteriole which supplies a variable number of capillaries which are drained by a venule. In some tissues the capillary network is short-circuited by an arteriovenous anastomosis. Pre- and post-capillary sphincters are shown; although only the former has been demonstrated histologically, indirect evidence suggests that there is also a post-capillary sphincter which reacts more slowly to the same factors that control the pre-capillary sphincter. The flow through the capillary bed is controlled by the hydrostatic pressure, the oncotic pressure and the sphincter tone. This is influenced by catecholamines and substances produced locally, which include carbon dioxide and hydrogen ion, accumulation of which causes the sphincters to relax. Local hypoxia has the same effect.

The vasomotor response

The four stages of the vasomotor response are indicated in Figure 5. Figure 5A shows the resting pattern, with the arteriovenous shunt closed and only one of the capillaries open. Figure 5B shows the first stage of the response to activation of the vasomotor centre. Vasoconstriction, which causes a rise in total peripheral resistance, is accompanied by cessation of capillary blood flow. The blood which flows through the arteriovenous shunt bypasses the tissues which become hypoxic and begin to suffer from autointoxication. At this stage prompt resuscitation will reverse these changes completely, but if not the pre-capillary sphincter opens while the post-capillary sphincter remains closed (Figure 5C). Blood enters the capillaries and stagnates. The hydrostatic pressure forces fluid and albumin out of the capillaries. The stagnant blood becomes hypoxic, hypercapnic and acidic, and other substances (bradykinin, prostaglandin $F_2\alpha$, etc.), some of which are mentioned later, accumulate. Intravascular coagulation may be initiated. In Figure 5D the post-capillary sphincter has finally relaxed, allowing the stagnant blood to re-enter the circulation carrying with it these metabolic waste products. By this time vulnerable organs such as the kidneys and liver will have been damaged. This is the second stage of shock.

Shock and the heart

The work done by the heart depends upon its rate and force of contraction and the total peripheral resistance, all of which are increased in the shocked patient. At the same time the coronary artery perfusion is reduced since this occurs principally during the diastolic interval, which is shortened by tachycardia. Young patients with good cardiac reserve should come to no harm in the short term, but the elderly or arteriopathic patient may quickly demonstrate clinical, biochemical and electrocardiographic signs of myocardial ischaemia. Cardiac enzymes, particularly the creatine phosphokinase, and the plasma lactate may rise to very high levels.

There is laboratory evidence which suggests that the venous blood which returns to the heart from ischaemic tissues contains vasodepressor materials which further reduce cardiac output.

Thus shock both increases the demands upon the heart and reduces its efficiency. This is the so-called 'vicious circle' mechanism.

Shock and the lung

This is discussed in detail in Chapter 5.

Shock and the kidneys

Under normal circumstances the kidneys receive approximately 20% of the total cardiac output, with 90% of this being distributed to the renal cortex. When the cardiac output or blood pressure fall, renal blood flow is correspondingly reduced and the urine output diminishes. As described above, the secretion of corticosteroids and ADH (vasopressin) are also involved. This process is readily reversed by adequate fluid replacement, but if it is allowed to persist, renal failure may develop.

If the patient has suffered burns or major crush injuries which involve soft tissues, hypotensive vasoconstriction may be aggravated by myoglobinuria. The relationship of myoglobin to renal failure is not clear, but there is good clinical evidence to support the thesis that muscle damage can cause renal failure in the absence of prolonged hypotension and vasoconstriction.

Shock may cause either acute tubular necrosis (ATN, acute 'reversible' renal failure) or acute cortical necrosis (acute 'irreversible' renal failure). Although this classification may appear to be clear-cut, the distinction between these conditions may sometimes be made only when the patient either regains or fails to regain renal function after an episode of acute renal failure, or at the autopsy.

Disseminated intravascular coagulation (DIC, consumption coagulopathy) may also be involved in the development of acute cortical necrosis. DIC occasionally follows uncomplicated trauma because of prolonged intravascular stasis, but more frequently it is associated with systemic sepsis; it may also follow an incompatible blood transfusion. The recognition of DIC is described on page 94.

Prognosis of acute renal failure

The prognosis for patients with acute tubular necrosis (ATN) is better than that for those with acute cortical necrosis, but this is partly dependent upon the patient's age. After an episode of ATN most patients who are less than 30 years of age should regain normal renal function, but the older the patient the less complete the degree of recovery. However, for many reasons—including the fact that they frequently have dysfunction of other organs (such as the lung)—the overall survival rate for patients whose injury is complicated by renal failure is still unsatisfactory. Only a very small minority of patients of any age who develop acute cortical necrosis can be expected to regain adequate renal function.

Recognition of acute renal failure

A patient is in renal failure when he fails to excrete enough urine to maintain fluid balance and to keep the plasma electrolyte, urea and creatinine levels within the normal limits. The volume of urine which is needed to achieve homeostasis is not constant; a patient who is normothermic and at rest need pass a much smaller volume than one who is pyrexial or has recently undergone major surgery or suffered multiple injuries. A figure of 30 ml/h is usually said to be adequate, but in the ITU even twice this amount may be insufficient.

The patient's renal function should be assessed daily during the acute phase of any illness so as to avoid the dangers of fluid and electrolyte overload. No individual test gives incontrovertible evidence, and it is usual for a battery of tests to be performed; however, if the plasma urea and creatinine levels are rising the patient is quite clearly not producing enough urine, whatever the cause may be. The tests which are listed in Table 1 should be carried out routinely. For the creatinine clearance to be measured, a 24-hour urine collection must be sent to the laboratory. The other tests can be performed on spot samples of blood and urine, although a 24-hour mean value is more reliable.

The ability to measure urine osmolality quickly and frequently is very useful, and a simple osmometer is a valuable piece of equipment in the ITU. The data it provides is not absolutely diagnostic, but when a patient has recently suffered physical injury or has had a major operation and is oliguric it is very helpful to be able to measure the urine osmolality and distinguish between pre-renal and intrinsic renal failure. The patient with pre-renal failure usually passes urine which has a high osmolality (more than 450 mosm/l),

Table 1. Renal function tests

Urine volume	At least 30 ml/h
$\dfrac{\text{Urine osmolality}}{\text{Blood osmolality}}$	$\dfrac{\text{At least 1.2}}{1}$
$\dfrac{\text{Urine urea}}{\text{Blood urea}}$	$\dfrac{\text{Greater than 13}}{1}$
Creatinine clearance	Greater than 30 1/24 h

whereas the patient with intrinsic renal failure almost always passes urine with an osmolality of less than 350 mosm/l.

Shock and the liver

The effects of shock upon hepatic function are less immediately apparent than are those upon the kidney, but they may carry an even worse prognosis.

Under normal circumstances the liver obtains 30% of its oxygen supply from the hepatic artery, the remainder being provided by the portal vein. It is easily damaged by hepatic arterial hypotension and by the effects of splanchnic vasoconstriction and stagnation, which cause the blood perfusing the liver to have an even lower oxygen content than usual. Splanchnic vasostagnation may also encourage the absorption of bacterial endotoxin from the gut, which may aggravate liver damage. Under normal circumstances endotoxin is destroyed by the hepatic reticuloendothelial system, but this is easily damaged by ischaemia and hypoxia.

If a battery of liver function tests is performed, including coagulation factors, clear evidence of hepatocellular damage may be obtained. If the serum amylase and lipase levels are measured at the same time, post-traumatic pancreatitis may also be recognized.

In the absence of biochemical tests, the first sign of liver damage is jaundice. This may be due to haemolysis of transfused blood or absorption of haematoma, and the bilirubin level often reaches very high levels indeed. The author recently had a patient whose bilirubin level ultimately reached 868 mmol/l due to absorption of haemoglobin from a retroperitoneal haematoma, which eventually caused abnormalities in hepatocellular function. The liver function tests returned to normal after 3 weeks.

Jaundice which is not caused by haemolysis has a very bad prognosis, usually because of its association with failure of other organs such as the lungs or kidneys and because of its relationship with systemic sepsis. Virtually every patient who has a major illness due to sepsis shows early signs of liver impairment.

Stress peptic ulceration

Stress peptic ulceration of the gastric or duodenal mucosa occurs in up to 10%

of patients who have suffered major trauma. This may manifest itself either as frank haematemesis or melaena, or more frequently by a progressive fall in the patient's haemoglobin level, which is explained by the finding of occult blood in the stool or gastric aspirate.

Stress peptic ulceration is particularly liable to occur in patients with a pre-existing history of peptic ulceration, but all are vulnerable. The causes are multiple, but they include increased gastric acidity due to stress and an increased plasma cortisol level, which reduces gastric mucosal resistance to autodigestion. There is also an increased secretion of gastrins, and patients who are in renal failure are particularly susceptible to stress peptic ulceration. Failure of the patient to take food by mouth reduces the neutralizing effect of foodstuffs against gastric acid. Although emotional stress may play a part, patients who are deeply sedated or unconscious for other reasons may develop stress ulceration. Every patient who has suffered a major physical insult should routinely be given an H_2 receptor blocker or regular antacids.

TRAUMA AND SEPSIS

A patient who has suffered a major injury is at risk from sepsis from two sources: (1) the injury itself, and (2) the treatment of the injury.

Major trauma reduces the body's resistance to infection by impairing the production of antibacterial antibody and complement and by reducing leucocyte mobility and phagocytosis. These effects are sustained by the high level of cortisol secretion. There is evidence that burned tissue produces a specific toxin which interferes with defence against infection.

The injury itself may increase the risk of infection. If the wound is grossly contaminated, or if the integrity of the gastrointestinal or genitourinary tracts is interrupted, an obvious source of systemic infection is created. Patients who have been immersed in polluted water are exposed to a similar hazard.

The treatment of many injuries involves the use of invasive techniques; these include surgical operations, but many of the procedures which are performed for resuscitative, monitoring or therapeutic purposes are only slightly less dangerous. Intravenous therapy, intravascular monitoring, endotracheal intubation, tracheostomy, chest drainage and the use of urinary catheters increase the hazard of local and systemic infection.

It is perhaps appropriate to point out that the anaesthetist is accustomed to deal with short-term emergencies such as asphyxia or severe haemorrhage, but many of the techniques he uses during resuscitation may have long-term and potentially harmful effects. He can minimize these by paying particular attention to asepsis, by being as gentle as possible in all his manoeuvres (such as intubation), and by using invasive monitoring techniques only when they are strictly necessary.

SEPTIC SHOCK

Septic shock is cardiocirculatory failure due either to an overwhelming bacterial infection or to a less severe bacteriological assault on a patient with reduced resistance. The term 'endotoxic shock' is less satisfactory since shock due to organisms which do not produce an endotoxin (e.g. *Staphylococcus aureus, Streptococcus pneumoniae*) is not materially different from that due to *Escherichia coli*.

The fundamental distinction between septic and haemorrhagic shock is that in the former the disturbance begins at cellular level and all of the tissues and organs are affected simultaneously, though not necessarily to the same degree, by the agents which cause the syndrome. Although the baroreceptors and the other components which were described earlier may be activated in septic shock, many additional factors are involved. Endotoxin is a lipopoly-saccharide which originates in the outer membranes of gram-negative bacteria such as *E. coli* and *Pseudomonas aeruginosa. Staphylococcus aureus* produces an alpha-haemolysin which may cause circulatory collapse. No comparable material has yet been identified from organisms such as *Streptococcus pneumoniae* or the meningococcus.

Other substances may be of secondary importance, arising directly or indirectly from damaged tissues, but they may help to perpetuate or complicate the disturbance. These include lysosomal breakdown products, vasodepressor material (VDM), bradykinin and other tissue kinins, throm-boxane, proteinases and prostaglandins. Serotonin and histamine released from damaged platelets undoubtedly play a part. Many of these substances are also released in phase 2 of haemorrhagic shock (Table 2).

Table 2. Factors involved in the development of septic shock

1. Pre-existing factor: diabetes, leukaemia, malignant disease
2. Extremes of age
3. Severity of injury, including burns and surgery
4. Abdominal or genitourinary tract involvement
5. Invasive monitoring
6. Intravenous therapy, including intravenous nutrition
7. Bladder catheterization, endotracheal intubation, tracheostomy, IPPV
8. Inappropriate antibiotic therapy
9. Immunosuppressive and corticosteroid drugs

Mode of presentation of septic shock

Septic shock most frequently develops in patients who are at risk because of the presence of sepsis in the abdomen, the genitourinary tract or elsewhere. It usually has an insidious onset, although occasionally it may present as sudden collapse during the course of urinary catheterization, bouginage, cystoscopy or similar procedures.

Hypotension, tachycardia and pyrexia are prominent features in most cases ('warm shock'); the degree of diastolic hypotension is disproportionate and in many cases the second Korotkof sound cannot be heard. This is a manifestation of gross peripheral vasodilatation and at this stage the patient's cardiac output is usually greatly elevated. Other signs include mental clouding, confusion, coma and occasionally, grand mal fits. In virtually every case oliguria occurs early and signs of renal impairment can be identified in the few non-oliguric patients. The relationship of shock, sepsis and jaundice has already been referred to.

Laboratory investigations usually demonstrate that in the early stages of septic shock the patient has a respiratory alkalaemia (hypocapnia) and mild hypoxia with an increased alveolar/arterial oxygen tension gradient (page 71). The arteriovenous oxygen tension difference is reduced, which indicates that the cardiac output is increased and also that tissue oxygen extraction is subnormal. If the condition does not respond to treatment, the patient usually goes on to develop a non-respiratory acidaemia with an elevated blood lactate and hypoxaemia which is resistant to all forms of oxygen therapy, together with the signs of multiple organ failure. Leucopenia, thrombocytopenia and disseminated intravascular coagulation (DIC) are common at this stage and are bad prognostic signs.

The small proportion of patients who die during the acute phase of septic shock pass from the stage of 'warm shock' to that of acute peripheral circulatory failure ('cold shock') which is resistant to treatment with blood volume expanders and pharmacological agents.

The 'capillary leak' syndrome

Within one to three days of its occurrence virtually every patient with septic shock shows some evidence of the 'capillary leak' syndrome. This is recognizable from the appearance of oedema of the face, limbs and flanks, and from radiographic evidence of interstitial pulmonary oedema, accompanied by hypoxaemia. This syndrome is presumed to be due to one or more of the substances, listed earlier, which increase capillary permeability by exerting an effect upon either the intercellular cement or the cell wall itself.

Endotoxin is too large a molecule to enter cells but it probably activates intermediary agents. It also increases the severity and duration of post-capillary veno-spasm, thus increasing the hydrostatic factor of the Starling equation (page 15) and aggravating the loss of fluid and albumin from the intravascular compartment into the tissues. Other studies have demonstrated that patients with septicaemia may lose up to 20% of their serum albumin in each 24 hours. Although this is partly due to diminished food intake and hypercatabolism, liver damage and loss of albumin into the interstitial tissues, particularly the lungs, are more important. The relationship of sepsis to acute respiratory failure is discussed in Chapter 5.

Other factors which are involved in the generation of oedema during the acute phase of resuscitation include fluid overload due to an unwise attempt to provoke a diuresis in the oliguric patient. Positive pressure ventilation not infrequently causes peri-orbital and conjunctival oedema.

Patients with shock due to sepsis may demonstrate clinical and laboratory signs of pancreatic damage, while patients with acute pancreatitis frequently develop septic shock. The high serum level of pancreatic enzymes and the correspondingly low serum calcium level are probably causative factors in the development of the capillary leak syndrome and of cardiac failure.

With standard methods of treatment, which are described later in this chapter, most patients with shock due to sepsis should survive the acute phase but up to 60% die days or weeks later from the combination of respiratory, renal and hepatic failure, together with chronic sepsis.

THE MONITORING AND TREATMENT OF HAEMORRHAGIC SHOCK

The most important feature of this condition is a reduction in the circulating blood volume due either to external or to occult losses. The special requirements of the burned patient are discussed in Chapter 7. Pain and the contribution made by myoglobin in the patient with crush injuries are referred to on page 17.

The first line of treatment is the replacement of the volume of fluid which has been lost. The factors which influence the choice of blood volume expanders have recently undergone a change of emphasis. Until ten years ago it was recommended that the correct treatment for blood loss was whole blood replacement, litre for litre. Estimates of the volume of blood required were based upon the concept that this could be predicted from the patient's clinical appearance. 'Mild' shock was said to be due to the loss of approximately 25% of the circulating blood volume, and in a previously fit patient the signs included tachycardia and peripheral vasoconstriction but with minimal change in the blood pressure. 'Severe' shock was said to result from the loss of up to 40% of the blood volume and the signs included pallor, tachycardia, hypotension, oliguria and peripheral vasoconstriction. Although this type of 'rule of thumb' assessment may be of some value, there is no doubt that the best indication of the volume of blood lost, unless this has been reliably measured, is the patient's response to fluid replacement.

Cardiocirculatory monitoring

The objectives of monitoring in the shocked patient are to recognize and record changes in organ and tissue perfusion and function as they occur. Many techniques are available, some of which can be used in unsophisticated establishments, whereas at the present time others are applicable only in a few of the most highly specialized research and treatment centres. In this section only the most basic methods will be described in any detail, although other more complex systems will be mentioned. Earlier, shock was defined in terms of organ and tissue failure; the monitoring of respiratory and renal function are referred to elsewhere in this book.

Minimal cardiocirculatory monitoring requires the recording of pulse rate and rhythm, the electrocardiograph pattern and the measurement of systemic blood pressure. Although intra-arterial monitoring is the most reliable and direct method, indirect ultrasonic or oscillotonometric methods are very satisfactory.

Essential investigations

Other fundamental investigations must be carried out. These include:
1   Core–skin temperature measurement

2   Urine output per hour and its osmolality
3   Central venous pressure in response to a fluid challenge
4   Blood gases, hydrogen ion status and alveolar/arterial oxygen tension gradient
5   Chest radiograph
6   Blood sugar
7   Plasma lactate
8   Cardiac enzymes
9   Serum amylase
10   Coagulation screen

Core–skin temperature measurement

The core temperature is recorded with a thermistor probe inserted into the external auditory canal, or in the oesophagus at 24 cm from the teeth. The skin temperature is measured on the dorsum or the hand or foot. The difference should not exceed 3°C unless the patient has been exposed to a low environmental temperature. If the gap is greater than 3°C, peripheral perfusion is probably reduced, usually because of hypovolaemia, and it should narrow in response to infusion. If the gap is greater than 3°C and the central venous pressure is high or rising, this is an indication for the use of alpha-adrenergic blocking drugs (discussed on page 36). Patients who are suffering from septicaemic shock do not usually have a wide core–skin temperature difference until the pre-terminal phase of the illness.

Central venous pressure monitoring

The central venous pressure level is a guide to right ventricular function, but only when measured in response to the fluid challenge. By itself it does not indicate the state of the circulating blood volume and the practice of 'filling up the CVP' to some pre-determined level should be abandoned. If the other indices of organ function are satisfactory, such as the core–skin temperature difference and the urine output, the CVP is acceptable. Evidence of overload, such as a triple rhythm audible at the apex of the heart or basal pulmonary crepitations, must constantly be guarded against.

The fluid challenge is performed as follows: 200 ml of a suitable fluid (PPF, Haemaccel, dextran) are infused over 15 minutes; if the CVP rises and does not return to its previous level after 15 minutes the infusion rate should be reduced. If the CVP rises but falls again to its previous level after 15 minutes, the central circulation can *probably* accept further fluid.

The other tests are performed for reasons which have been outlined elsewhere. It is essential to identify deterioration in respiratory function as soon as it develops, since this may be an indication for the use of diuretics or for the administration of oxygen or IPPV with or without PEEP. The methods used include the frequent measurement of blood gases and the Aa oxygen tension gradient (page 71) together with chest radiography. The blood sugar level should be maintained at the upper limit of normal throughout this critical period to provide a readily available source of calories.

Additional data

In all but the most complex cases, the monitoring methods described above will provide all the information which is necessary for treatment to be applied. More sophisticated and less essential information may be provided by pulmonary wedge pressure measurement and cardiac output determination.

Pulmonary wedge pressure measurement

With flow-directed balloon catheters the pulmonary wedge pressure can easily be measured. It provides information about the function of the left ventricle which should be taken together with CVP measurement, urine output and core–skin temperature measurement to indicate when fluid restriction or inotropic agents such as dopamine should be used. The normal pressure range is 15–20 mm Hg, and if it rises above this level during resuscitation, the probability of overload or of left ventricular failure exists. If pulmonary oedema occurs at a pressure lower than 15 mm Hg, ARDS or hypoalbuminaemia are the likely causes.

When multifunction balloon catheters are used, the cardiac output can be calculated by the thermal dilution method and mixed venous blood obtained, so that tissue oxygen extraction can be calculated. This is of particular value in septicaemic shock, when the arteriovenous oxygen tension difference is often less than would be expected from the raised cardiac output, which demonstrates poor oxygen extraction by damaged tissues.

Possession of these additional data is unlikely to make a vital difference to the treatment of shocked patients, although PWP monitoring is useful in the diagnosis and treatment of cardiogenic shock.

All forms of invasive monitoring create potential hazards, but the risks from pulmonary wedge pressure monitoring are higher than those which accompany CVP monitoring. When the balloon is inflated, up to 15% of the blood supply of the lung is occluded. This is obviously undesirable, and the balloon should be deflated immediately after each measurement has been made. Further complications of this investigation are reported frequently. In addition to local and systemic infection, these include pulmonary infarction, haemorrhage, knotting of the catheter leading to difficulty with withdrawal, cardiac rupture, tamponade and many dysrhythmias. It is probable that in the near future this method of monitoring will be replaced by one or other of the two discussed below.

Aortovelography

This technique is used to measure cardiac output by the reflection of ultrasound from blood flowing through the aortic arch. It is completely non-invasive and simple to use and appears to give results which are at least as good as those obtained by other means. If its value is substantiated it will become a useful addition to the other methods used at the present time.

Radionuclide imaging

This method is based upon the computer-aided visualization of the distribution of suitable tracers through the heart and pulmonary circulation. It can be used to demonstrate heart shape and size and, in particular, the completeness of cardiac emptying and the position of the interventricular septum. At the present time this is a research tool and its cost makes it likely to remain so for the foreseeable future.

Volume replacement

The importance of replacing blood which is lost with an equivalent volume of whole blood has been reviewed. It is now generally accepted that a haemoglobin level of 10 g/dl and a haematocrit of 35% are quite adequate and may confer positive benefits through economy in blood usage, by reducing the recipient's blood viscosity, and by improving tissue blood flow. It may also reduce the incidence of post-traumatic thromboembolic episodes. If a patient has a fixed cardiac output, or has ischaemic heart disease, the effects of any degree of haemodilution must be carefully monitored since it may lead to a demand for an increased cardiac output which the heart cannot satisfy.

The overtransfusion hazard

The argument as to whether colloidal fluids are better than crystalloids for emergency resuscitation is not yet settled. Several authors have presented opposing views which are based upon clinical and experimental investigations. At present the evidence suggests that if the patient has normal renal function, it may be less dangerous to overtransfuse him with crystalloid than with colloid, since the latter seems more likely to cause persistent overload and pulmonary oedema. However, provided that overload is avoided, colloid solutions have other advantages which are discussed later in this section.

Buffered sodium lactate solutions (Ringer's, Hartmann's) are widely used during resuscitation and when given as part of a balanced regime they are useful. However, early enthusiasm for this type of solution ('white blood') has waned since it was recognized that overenthusiastic infusion was a major cause of respiratory difficulties in the traumatized patient ('Da Nang Wet Lung', shock lung, ARDS, etc.) (Chapter 5).

Until relatively recently overtransfusion was almost unknown, but this is no longer the case. Although where doubt exists a moderate degree of overtransfusion is better than gross undertransfusion, many patients who have undergone vigorous emergency resuscitation are subsequently found to have pulmonary oedema. The intermediate stage treatment of the shocked patient often includes fluid restriction and the use of diuretics such as frusemide.

Oxygen transport and coagulation

Other than blood, no intravenous solution in general use has oxygen-carrying capability, although fluorocarbon solutions and stroma-free haemoglobin have been used for this purpose on a small scale and are soon to be more freely available.

The effects of massive blood volume replacement upon blood coagulation must be considered. Poor wound healing and the occurrence of spontaneous bleeding from the respiratory, gastrointestinal and genitourinary tracts may be attributed to ill-judged replacement of coagulation factors.

General guidelines to volume replacement

With these and other provisos borne in mind, guidelines to intravenous fluid replacement for the traumatized patient can be given.

1 In an emergency any blood volume expander is better than none.

2 A 'normal' haemoglobin level is not essential to life, and blood transfusions should be given only as part of a balanced infusion regimen to maintain the haemoglobin and haematocrit levels at or near the values suggested above.

3 All infusions which are not in category 1 above should be regarded as dangerous drugs with potentially undesirable side-effects which therefore should be *prescribed* after due thought.

4 In addition to their desirable and evanescent qualities as blood volume expanders, their biochemical, pharmacological, haematological and allergic/toxic properties should be considered.

Some of the properties of the infusion fluids which are most frequently used are shown in Table 3.

When any blood volume expander is prescribed, the factors which should be considered are:

1 Safety, including allergenicity
2 Compatibility with other IV fluids
3 Duration of stay in the circulation
4 Positive benefits, e.g. haemoglobin, albumin, coagulation factors
5 Interference with cross-matching and blood coagulation
6 Cost
7 Availability

Most intravenous fluids have a wide safety margin and they should all be bacteriologically sterile. However, they may be contaminated either in preparation or in storage, and septicaemic episodes which are otherwise inexplicable may be traced to this source. Bacterial contamination is most frequently caused by the addition of substances to the container in the ward. Some intravenous fluids are very good culture media and nothing should ever be added to packs containing blood or blood products.

Infusion reactions

Up to 5% of the recipients of blood transfusion can be expected to suffer a reaction, but this is usually trivial unless the blood transfusion service or the doctor administering the infusion has made a mistake with identification. Most reactions are caused by protein sensitization and, except when incompatible blood has been infused, investigation rarely reveals any cause in

Table 3. Commonly used infusion fluids

	Blood	PPF	Dextran 40	Dextran 70	Gelatine products	HES
Availability	Variable	Variable	Good	Good	Good	Variable
Cost	High	High	Modest	Modest	Modest	High
Hepatitis risk	Present	Absent	—	—	—	?
Allergenicity	Present	Rare	+	++	+	—
Microembolism risk	Present	—	—	—	—	—
Oxygen carriage	Yes, but varies	No	No	No	No	No
Albumin content	30g/l	30g/l	—	—	—	—
Duration of action as blood volume expander	24 h	12 h	2 h	4 h	2 h	24 h +
Sodium	140 mmol/l	140 mmol/l	Available in normal saline or dextrose		—	140 mmol/l
Potassium	3–4 mmol/l up to 20 mmol/l	2.2–2.4 mmol/l			—	—
Calcium	0.5–1.5 mmol/l	—	—	—	3–4 mmol/l	—
Special problems	Microaggregates 2,3-DPG, etc	—	May cause renal damage	Cross-match problems	Immiscible with blood	Cross-match problems

the donor, the blood pack or the recipient. Haemolytic transfusion reactions can cause DIC and acute renal failure. In the United Kingdom blood donors are routinely checked to minimize the risk of transmission of hepatitis B antigen and this should be a very uncommon complication of blood transfusion. In some other countries the risk is still quite high.

Reactions to plasma protein factor (PPF, human albumin in saline solution) are most unusual.

Dextran 70 is a useful blood volume expander, but allergic reactions—which vary in severity from minor skin reactions to bronchospasm and cardiocirculatory collapse—are said to occur in about 1 in 1000 units infused. Haemaccel and Gelofusine have not been available long enough for a full assessment to be made, although it appears that sensitivity reactions to these agents occur at least as frequently as with the dextrans. Haemaccel contains 3.13 mmol calcium ions per litre. If blood is infused simultaneously through a Y-connection, or subsequently through the same giving set, clots may form which will either block the set or, rarely, be infused into the patient. If blood is to be transfused after Haemaccel the giving set should be changed.

Many blood transfusion services use sophisticated methods of plasma separation and fractionation, and as a consequence up to 80% of the blood held in blood banks is either plasma-reduced or is packed red cells. The patient should be given the appropriate volume of a plasma volume expander together with packed cells in order to maintain the circulating blood volume.

Disadvantages of blood transfusion

Blood appears to be the ideal infusion fluid for patients who have suffered major blood volume loss, but in an earlier section this was questioned. It has been emphasized that when large volumes of blood are lost (more than 30% of the circulating blood volume) blood should form part of the infusion regime. The problems which may result from the transfusion of stored blood can be considered under six headings, some of which have already been mentioned. These are:

1 Availability and cost
2 Collection and storage problems
3 Physical effects of transfusion
4 Biochemical problems
5 Coagulation factors
6 Incompatibility and sensitivity reactions

Some of the problems which follow blood transfusion are aggravated with increasing age of the stored blood. At present, blood is returned to the transfusion service after it has been stored for 21 days, but advances in preservation, suspension and storage methods can be expected to extend its storage life. These include the use of deep-frozen and resuspended red cells and the addition of adenosine triphosphate or glycerol to the preservative. At present, these techniques are used only by a minority of transfusion services and the problems which are described in this section still exist.

Availability and cost

Blood for transfusion should be regarded as a precious commodity to be used only when strictly necessary. In the field only small quantities of Group O rhesus-negative blood are likely to be available, and blood may be in short supply in hospital. This is not always related to the blood group, and blood of an unusual group may be more freely available than that of a more common group since the former is, by definition, less frequently required.

No realistic price tag can be attached to a unit of blood. Figures ranging from £40 to £50 per unit are quoted, but in the United Kingdom donors are not paid and the cost is related to the efficiency of the blood transfusion service and its irreducible overheads.

Collection and storage problems

The selection of donors should minimize the hazard of transmissible diseases such as hepatitis and syphilis. Donors who have recently taken drugs such as aspirin or penicillin, which may cause allergic reactions in the recipient, should be rejected.

Donor blood is collected into packs which contain an anticoagulant—either acid citrate dextrose (ACD) or citrate phosphate dextrose (CPD), both of which act by combining with calcium ions. Platelets and 2,3-diphosphogly-cerate are better preserved by CPD anticoagulant, but in either case most platelets disappear within 24 hours of blood donation. Other coagulation factors are lost more slowly, but after five days in the bank no significant coagulant qualities remain.

ACD (120 ml) or CPD (75 ml) is added to each unit of blood at the time of collection, so each unit has only 75–80% of the haemoglobin content of the donor. While in storage, the red cells gradually lyse and the haemoglobin content of 21-day-old blood is generally less than 10 g/dl. The plasma haemoglobin level rises commensurately.

Citrate intoxication

It is often stated that when large volumes of ACD blood are transfused the recipient may show signs of citrate intoxication. These include depression of cardiac output, a bleeding tendency and, rarely, tetany; occasionally the recipient complains of a tingling sensation around the mouth. These features are said to be due to hypocalcaemia. The likelihood of serious problems being created is remote, since the body's calcium stores are large and the immediate effect of a large volume transfusion is a transient acidaemia which tends to increase the ionized calcium level. However, many anaesthetists routinely give calcium supplements to patients who are receiving large volume transfusions. Calcium chloride is usually given at an arbitrary rate of 5 ml 10% solution for every 3 l blood infused. It should not be injected into a central line since this may cause bradycardia of asystole. Obviously, it must not be injected into the infusion line through which the blood is given.

Potassium

During storage, potassium leaks out of the red cells into the plasma, and at the end of 21 days in storage the plasma potassium level may be as high as 20.0 mmol/l. In the average patient this should not matter, but if a patient with renal impairment receives a large volume transfusion of 21-day-old blood he may develop the signs of hyperkalaemia.

Hydrogen ion effects

The pH of blood changes from 7.4 at the time of donation to between 6.8 and 7.0 at the time of its infusion, depending upon its age. This is in part due to the pH of the anticoagulant (6.5) and in part to the continued metabolic activity of the cells during storage. Immediately after the blood is reinfused there is a transient fall in the recipient's plasma pH (non-respiratory acidaemia), the degree of which depends upon the age, volume and rate of reinfusion and upon the buffering capacity of the recipient's blood. However, within 2–4 hours of the infusion being completed the patient usually develops a non-respiratory alkalaemia through the metabolism of the citrate anticoagulant to bicarbonate. This may persist for 24–48 hours after the transfusion is completed, and it is the usual cause of the non-respiratory alkalaemia which is commonly noted on the first day after transfusion.

Microaggregates and filtration

Red cells, platelets and leucocytes undergo denaturation in storage and may aggregate into debris which can pass through the standard infusion filter. Albumin and fibrinogen may be included in the aggregate. At present, interest is concentrated on the possibility that this debris is filtered by the recipient's pulmonary capillaries, perhaps to become a factor in the development of post-traumatic respiratory insufficiency (adult respiratory distress syndrome, shock lung, etc.). Leucocyte debris is thought to be particularly important because of the vasoactive material it releases.

A wide variety of infusion microfilters is now available with pore sizes of 20–40 μm. Although the evidence that they are necessary is hard to evaluate, many experienced clinicians feel they should be used when large volumes of blood are being transfused rapidly (more than 1 l/h). Since a 'best buy' cannot be recommended on scientific grounds, it is sensible to use the filter which will allow the unimpeded flow of the largest volume of blood at the lowest cost to the exchequer. Filtration removes the debris which is large enough to be filtered by and obstruct the pulmonary capillaries. However, platelets and white cells which are filtered out before the blood reaches the patient may still release vasoactive amines such as histamine and serotonin (5-hydroxytrypt-amine). The microfilter must be removed from the infusion set if blood is to be followed by electrolyte solutions, dextran or similar substances since these can 'wash through' the material deposited upon the filter.

Oxygen carriage

The oxygen-carrying capacity of blood depends upon the number of intact red cells, their haemoglobin content (and its type) and the quantity of the enzyme 2,3-diphosphoglycerate (2,3-DPG) present inside the red cells. The effects upon the cell population of dilution and storage have already been referred to. The red cell 2,3-DPG falls during storage, causing the haemoglobin's affinity for oxygen to increase and reducing its availability to the tissues. This is partly corrected by rewarming the blood during infusion and restored completely within 12 hours of infusion, but until such time the oxygen-delivering capacity of the transfused blood is reduced.

Cooling

Banked blood is stored at 4°C to reduce cell metabolism and the rate of replication of any bacteria which may have been introduced at the time of its donation. If large volumes of cold blood are infused the patient will inevitably be cooled, and if he is conscious he will complain or begin to shiver. If the blood is infused through a peripheral vein this will go into spasm and slow the infusion rate. If it is infused rapidly through a central line it is remotely possible that cardiac slowing or ventricular dysrhythmias may ensue.

　　Various types of blood-warming device are available although none is suitable for use in the field. Several cases of septicaemia have been attributed to the use of coils immersed in water baths, and at the present time some type of dry-block warming system is probably to be preferred. This should be capable of warming blood from its storage temperature to 36–37°C when infused at a rate of 5 l/h. In addition to its effects upon 2,3-DPG rewarming encourages the return of potassium into red cells. It is probable that the metabolism of citrate to bicarbonate by the liver is hastened if the patient's core temperature is maintained.

Coagulation factors

Stored blood contains no useful amounts of clotting factors, and patients who have received large volume transfusions may show signs of bleeding. In most cases this is due to the trauma itself or to surgery, and no less obvious cause need be sought. Rarely, DIC may be found to be the cause, and occasionally a shortage of coagulation factors may be incriminated. Platelet synthesis is very efficient, and 24 hours after an exchange transfusion the platelet level is usually found to be adequate (more than $60\,000/mm^{-3}$). This degree of thrombocytopenia may be more significant if it is due to sepsis or to drugs.

　　The recipient's other coagulation factors are inevitably lowered by dilution, although it is hard to define levels at which replacements should be given. Not all patients who have the same degree of lowering of coagulation factors bleed from surgical wounds or elsewhere.

　　Fresh frozen plasma (FFP) contains fibrinogen (Factor I) and the prothrombin complex (Factors II, VII, IX, X). Patients who are receiving large volume transfusions are often given one pack of FFP to every 3 l blood given. The effects of this practice are hard to evaluate, but since FFP is itself a good blood volume expander with few side-effects its use in this way can only be beneficial—unless it reduces its availability for patients whose need is more obvious.

Platelet concentrate may also be used, but again its effects are difficult to assess. After the administration of many units of platelets the recipient's platelet count rarely rises dramatically. With techniques available at present platelets cannot be completely separated from red cells and only ABO compatible platelets can be used. The half-life of transfused platelets is approximately 24 hours. They should not be given through microfilters since large numbers of both normal and clumped platelets will be trapped by the filter. If a patient shows signs of abnormal bleeding—as for example from previously healed wounds, from venipuncture sites, or internally—and the platelet count is less than $40\,000/mm^{-3}$, platelet infusions may be given. Thrombocytopenia without bleeding is not an indication for platelet transfusion but, as suggested earlier, it may be an ominous sign in the septicaemic patient.

Plasma protein fraction (PPF)

This is 4.5% human albumin in saline together with small amounts of alpha- and beta-globulin; 25% albumin (low salt) is also available but this is not intended to be used in resuscitation.

PPF is the ideal blood volume expander if oxygen transport is not required. In preparation it is heated to 60°C for 10 hours to inactivate hepatitis virus. It can be stored at room temperature (between 2°C and 25°C) for up to 5 years provided that it is protected from direct sunlight. Allergic reactions are extremely uncommon.

After infusion a useful amount remains in the circulation for up to 24 hours. Thereafter it is metabolized and enters the amino acid pool. In addition to being an effective blood volume expander, it contributes to the plasma oncotic pressure and may improve the microvascular circulation.

Albumin infusions frequently cause a diuresis and when the first stage of resuscitation is completed, PPF may be given to aid the mobilization of intrapulmonary water. Its use in the treatment of the adult respiratory distress syndrome is described in Chapter 5.

Dextran solutions

In Britain three dextran preparations are used clinically, classified according to their mean molecular weight:
    Dextran 110 (000)—high molecular weight
    Dextran   70 (000)—medium molecular weight
    Dextran   40 (000)—low molecular weight

All three are available in either normal saline or 5% dextrose. Dextran 40 is rapidly excreted in urine and is not used as a blood volume expander; if the patient's renal function is impaired, Dextran 40 may cause further deterioration. It is possible that Dextran 70 may also cause renal tubular damage, although if so this is very uncommon.

Dextran 70 is a good blood volume expander. About 20% is excreted within three hours of infusion, but a significant fraction remains in the circulation for up to six hours. Through its effect upon oncotic pressure it increases the plasma volume indirectly by causing a shift of interstitial water into the intravascular compartment. In Britain, high molecular weight dextrans (110 000 or 250 000) are rarely used. Allergic reactions to dextrans occur with increasing frequency in parallel with their molecular weight.

By reducing platelet adhesiveness, dextrans may interfere with blood coagulation and increase post-traumatic and post-operative bleeding. They may also make subsequent cross-matching difficult. It is usually recommended that only one litre of dextran should be given in any 24-hour period because of these effects; on the other hand they may also reduce the risks of post-operative and post-traumatic thromboembolism.

Any dextran molecules which are not excreted in the urine are metabolized to carbon dioxide and water.

Gelatin solutions

Several gelatin preparations are available. They all have similar properties and only two are described here.

Haemaccel This is a 3.5% solution of mean molecular weight 40 000 and pH 7.1. It can be stored at room temperature for up to 5 years. Because some of the material has a molecular weight below the renal threshold (30 000) it is excreted in the urine within 2 hours. Small amounts may be retained by the reticuloendothelial system for up to 48 hours.

Allergic reactions are uncommon, and none of the presently used gelatin preparations interfere with blood cross-matching, which means they can be given at the site of an accident without worrying about the consequences. Haemaccel contains relatively large amounts of calcium which may cause clotting in infusion sets if it is given sequentially with blood.

Gelofusine This is 3% modified fluid gelatin (MFG) with a mean molecular weight of 35 000 and pH 5.8. In other respects it is similar to Haemaccel but contains less calcium.

It was stated above that only one litre of dextran should be given in any 24-hour period. In contrast, many litres of gelatin solutions can be given, without apparent harm, provided that the patient has normal renal function.

Hydroxyethyl starch (HES)

This substance was first used in 1957. It is available in 6% solution and has many features in common with Dextran 110. Its properties have been widely investigated in Japan, but it has not been extensively used in Britain. It appears to have few toxic side-effects but anxiety has been expressed about its ultimate fate in the body since it may stay in the circulation for a prolonged period. In experimental animals HES has been found in the reticuloendothelial system many days after infusion, which may interfere with protection against infection. Blood should be taken for cross-matching before HES is given.

The choice of blood volume expander

From the data given in the above section it is apparent that a wide variety of fluids is available for resuscitation, and recommendations can only be based upon the extensive literature on the subject combined with personal experience. Most clinicians share the opinion that PPF is the best volume expander when given together with sufficient blood to maintain the patient's haemoglobin level at around 10 g/dl. If PPF is not available, gelatin solutions are second choice. Gelatin may be used as first choice when short-term infusion therapy is required by a patient who was previously physically fit, or when the serum albumin level is not critically reduced. Examples of these situations include the treatment of a brisk external haemorrhage of up to one litre which can be expected to stop abruptly with treatment, or a closed femoral shaft fracture. Dextran 70 is third in order of preference because of the relatively high incidence of allergic reactions which occur and its possible nephrotoxicity. Dextran 70 may cause an unacceptable shift of transcellular water into the circulating blood as its colloid osmotic pressure is greater than that of plasma. Theoretically this could cause secondary loss of intracellular fluid and interfere with the function of tissues, including cardiac and voluntary muscle.

Plasma protein synthesis by the liver is regulated by the oncotic pressure in the hepatic interstitium. All artificial colloids (dextrans, gelatin, HES, etc.) inhibit the hepatic synthesis of albumin in proportion to and for the duration of their intravascular oncotic effect; these substances should therefore not be used as substitutes for albumin.

The use of pharmacological agents in haemorrhagic shock

In most cases, restoration of the circulating blood volume is all that is required. However, it may occasionally be necessary to use catecholamines and drugs which improve peripheral blood flow.

Dopamine

If a patient becomes oliguric at any stage during resuscitation the urine osmolality should be measured. If it is greater than 500 mmol/l the patient probably needs more fluid. However, if the other observations suggest that the patient has had an adequate infusion a dopamine infusion should be set up. Dopamine stimulates both alpha- and beta-adrenoreceptors, but its effects upon the renal dopaminergic receptors are often more useful. It is a very safe drug and it should be used early rather than late. When given at the rate of 2–6 μg/kg/min it has minimal effects upon pulse rate and rhythm or blood pressure, but it improves renal blood flow and often causes a notable diuresis in the shocked patient; its use may reduce the risk of acute renal failure.

Dopamine infusion should be given by syringe pump or a similar device and it should always be infused through a central line because, if it extravasates, its alpha-stimulant effects predominate and it can cause extensive tissue necrosis.

Dobutamine

Dobutamine is primarily a beta-1 agonist which improves cardiac output by increasing the stroke volume. It has almost no effect upon heart rate and rhythm and, because its alpha stimulant effects are trivial, it can safely be given through a peripheral vein if necessary. The recommended dose ranges from 2.5 to 10 μg/kg/min. It has no specific effects on renal blood flow but may cause a diuresis through increasing the cardiac output. It may be given together with dopamine in the early stages of treatment of septicaemic shock, although this type of polypharmacy should be used only when strictly necessary.

Isoprenaline

Isoprenaline is a beta-1 agonist but it has beta-2 effects which may be very useful in the treatment of status asthmaticus. It usually causes a tachycardia and may cause other tachydysrhythmias. In addition to its effects on the peripheral circulation it reduces pulmonary arteriolar pressure. It has no specific beneficial effects upon renal perfusion. It is given by infusion at the rate of 0.05 μg/kg/min.

The use of diuretics

Neither frusemide nor similar diuretics are helpful in the shocked patient unless he shows signs of left ventricular failure or interstitial pulmonary oedema. Diuretics are not therapeutic agents; they do not cure acute renal failure and there is no evidence that they protect the patient against impending renal damage.

Mannitol is a very effective osmotic diuretic which may be useful, for example, in the jaundiced patient with moderately severe renal impairment. However, since it is also an osmotic blood volume expander it should not be given to the patient who is volume-overloaded since it may precipitate him into heart failure.

Alpha-adrenergic blockade

The best peripheral vasodilator is an adequate circulating blood volume, but a patient who has been in peripheral circulatory failure for more than 1 or 2 hours may not respond immediately to simple blood volume replacement. The periphery may remain cold and blue in spite of a rising central venous pressure. These signs are the indications for the use of alpha-adrenergic blocking agents. Phenoxybenzamine and thymoxamine are the best known members of this group of drugs but they may be too powerful or too long-lasting. Phenoxybenzamine is usually given by infusion at the rate of 10 mg/kg/h after an initial loading dose of 0.5 mg/kg. The results are monitored as described later in this chapter, but include core-to-skin temperature measurement. Phenoxybenzamine has a duration of action of 6 to 8 hours and its actions cannot be reversed.

Thymoxamine may be given as a bolus injection 0.5–1.0 mg/kg body weight. Its effects are much less dramatic than phenoxybenzamine and last 30 to 60 minutes. Although this is rarely necessary, if it is felt that its effects need to be reversed, a dopamine infusion at the rate 10–15 μg/kg/min may be given.

For several years the author has used chlorpromazine as an effective vasodilator in the dose range 5–25 mg intravenously. Its alpha-blocking effects are demonstrated by an improvement in the patient's skin colour and by a narrowing of the core–skin temperature difference.

Chlorpromazine and specific alpha-adrenergic blockers must not be given until the patient has been adequately transfused, as demonstrated by his fluid balance chart, with generous allowance for occult losses. The central venous pressure and/or pulmonary wedge pressure must be high. Although serious adverse reactions to chlorpromazine are rare, they can be anticipated if thymoxamine or phenoxybenzamine are given to a patient with a shrunken blood volume.

Alpha-stimulant drugs (methoxamine, noradrenaline, metaraminol, methyl amphetamine, etc.) and corticosteroids are never used in the treatment of either haemorrhagic or septicaemic shock.

THE TREATMENT OF SEPTICAEMIC SHOCK

The principles that govern the treatment of this condition are:
1 Maintenance of the circulating blood volume
2 Support of organ function
3 Control of the underlying infection

Volume replacement

Many patients who develop the signs of septicaemic shock are already hypovolaemic and this must be corrected; others may appear to require large volume transfusions without having lost much fluid externally. This is the main feature of the capillary leak syndrome. Monitoring was described earlier, but in addition the haematocrit must be measured every 3 to 6 hours during resuscitation as a guide to plasma losses. If the haematocrit rises during resuscitation, it indicates that capillary leakage has begun, or that fluid is being lost into closed compartments such as the pleural or peritoneal cavity. Systemic and pulmonary oedema are prominent features of septicaemia; this must be constantly borne in mind and overtransfusion avoided at all costs.

Choice of volume expander

PPF is the first-choice plasma volume expander, although whole blood may also be required. Unless the plasma albumin level is monitored daily and the appropriate treatment given, the level may drop by up to 20% each 24 hours. Even when albumin supplements are given the level may fall below 30 g/l and albumin is probably lost through leaky capillaries into the lungs and elsewhere. The use of albumin solutions in the septicaemic patient has been criticized on the basis that they may aggravate rather than prevent or reduce interstitial pulmonary oedema. This is a difficult problem, but at present it appears to be more logical to use oncotically active agents (colloids) than crystalloids in this situation.

Use of digoxin and other agents

Both experimental and clinical evidence indicate that every patient with septicaemia should be digitalized. Because of the high incidence of renal impairment the plasma digoxin level should be monitored after two days of treatment with this drug. The place of prostaglandin inhibitors is discussed in Chapter 5.

The use of dopamine in the shocked patient was described earlier. The indications for its use in septicaemia are similar to those already given, although it may also be used in a higher dose (up to 10 μg/kg/min) to support the systemic circulation. This dose rate may have alpha-stimulant effects; if so it should be reduced and given together with dobutamine. When the patient's condition has stabilized the dopamine infusion should be discontinued abruptly. There is nothing to be gained by reducing the dose by degrees, and many patients develop an apparently paradoxical rise in arterial blood pressure 15 to 20 minutes after the drug has been discontinued.

Occasionally a patient in shock due to sepsis is found to have a low ionized calcium level (when corrected for the serum albumin). Although this is of doubtful significance, rarely, calcium chloride injection may bring about an improvement in cardiocirculatory function.

Controlled ventilation in septicaemic shock

Of all forms of treatment of septicaemic shock, none has so much improved the prognosis of what is still a lethal condition as the early institution of controlled ventilation. Septicaemia is always associated with a widening of the alveolar–arterial oxygen tension gradient and if it progresses, absolute hypoxia is inevitable, leading to irreversible damage to the kidneys, liver and other organs. This condition is discussed in greater detail in Chapter 5, but every patient with septicaemia should be admitted to the Intensive Therapy Unit, intubated and ventilated with oxygen-enriched air. The indications for this treatment include clinical and radiographic evidence of atelectasis with an arterial oxygen tension of less than 7 kPa, when the patient is breathing room air. The causes of respiratory failure in septicaemic patients are listed in Table 4.

Controlled ventilation is initially applied via an endotracheal tube but later it may be necessary to perform a tracheostomy. Only enough additional oxygen should be used to maintain an acceptable arterial oxygen tension (more than 8 kPa). Other aspects of controlled ventilation in the septicaemic patient, including the use of PEEP, are discussed in Chapter 5.

Septicaemia and the 'sick cell syndrome'

Many septicaemic patients are hyponatraemic. This is usually caused by inappropriate intravenous therapy and its resultant haemodilution, but the 'sick cell syndrome' is occasionally responsible. This is caused by generalized

Table 4. Reasons for respiratory failure in the septicaemic patient

Fluid overload

Atelectasis

Bronchopneumonia

Hypoproteinaemia

Pulmonary microembolism/microthrombosis/ARDS

Interstitial oedema

Increased metabolic rate/oxygen consumption

Reduced efficiency of the respiratory muscles

Ventilation/perfusion imbalance

Increased alveolar dead space

Intra-abdominal sepsis and diaphragmatic splinting

cell damage and, in addition to its occurrence in septicaemia, it may also be identified in patients with burns, congestive cardiac failure, severe pneumonia, and poisoning with some drugs, including alcohol. It results from cell wall damage accompanied by failure of intracellular metabolic processes, particularly the sodium pump. As a consequence sodium and water accumulate within cells and potassium and organic phosphates leak out. Cardiac failure, pulmonary oedema and oliguria commonly result; the renal excretion of sodium falls, and if sodium balance studies are carried out it becomes apparent that the whole body sodium content is rising.

The diagnosis of the sick cell syndrome is made by comparing the actual plasma osmolality when measured directly with the value obtained by adding together the individual parts of the laboratory electrolyte screen. As an example:

Actual osmolality:		295 mmol/l
Calculated osmolality:	Sodium	125 ($\times$ 2) mmol/l
	Potassium	4.0 ($\times$ 2) mmol/l
	Urea	4.0 mmol/l
	Glucose	5.0 mmol/l
	Creatinine Calcium Magnesium Phosphate Sulphate	say 5 mmol/l
	Total	272 mmol/l

The discrepancy of 23 mmol/l is greater than that which can be explained by minor ions and should suggest the diagnosis of sick cell syndrome.

Treatment of the sick cell syndrome

At present the treatment of this condition is empirical. Insulin is the only agent readily available which can stimulate intracellular activity, although adenosine triphosphate (ATP) has also been used for this purpose. Usually, a glucose and insulin infusion is set up (20 units of insulin, 50 g glucose) and administered over four hours. This is repeated so that up to 120 units of insulin are given in each 24 hours. It is usually necessary to give additional potassium to maintain normal levels. The beneficial effects of treatment are shown by an improvement in the patient's cardiac output and a rise in the serum sodium, together with an increase in the urinary water and sodium excretion.

Patients with the 'sick cell syndrome' should not be given sodium infusions since the sodium accumulates inside cells and increases the intracellular volume, which aggravates tissue damage and organ failure. The heart is particularly vulnerable to intracellular sodium and water accumulation.

Control of the underlying infection

This is the most difficult part of treatment. The factors which are associated with septicaemia are set out in Table 4. Although these include the primary cause, many of them are inseparable from its treatment, including the use of intravenous and intra-arterial lines, endotracheal intubation, and IPPV and urinary catheterization. In many cases these cannot be dispensed with, but every form of invasive treatment or monitoring must be balanced against its possible side-effects and discontinued as soon as possible. Intravenous catheters, such as those used for CVP measurement or parenteral nutrition, should be removed, even if only for 24 hours, until an adequate blood antibiotic level is achieved. They can then be reinserted at a different site. Long lines should not be used as injection points since this probably increases the risk of secondary infection. Arterial lines should not be left in place for more than 72 hours.

Re-exploration

In many cases the source of the infection may be suspected (e.g., subphrenic abscess or other localized collection) and identified by ultrasound or the gallium scan. Unfortunately many surgeons are unwilling to re-operate upon patients with septicaemia through fear of anaesthetic complications. The anaesthetist must recognize that in many cases only re-exploration and drainage of sources of infection can allow the patient to survive, and he must be prepared to anaesthetize any patient for whom such treatment offers some hope. Exploration may need to be repeated on several occasions, but fear of the coroner must never be allowed to influence a decision which is clinically correct. A more important consideration is the opinion of the patient's relatives; they must be kept fully aware of the reasons for re-operation, and informed of the possible consequences.

Choice of antibiotics

The choice of antibiotic treatment for the septicaemic patient is not wide. In many cases this is dictated by microbiological evidence obtained before the patient became acutely ill: for example, *Escherichia coli* or *Klebsiella* sp. may have been identified in specimens taken at the first operation, or grown from subsequent sputum, drainage or urine samples. Many hospitals have an antibiotic policy which is designed to deal with all eventualities and which is partly dependent upon known hospital organisms. It is not possible, therefore, to make absolute recommendations for treatment. The author uses a balanced broad spectrum combination as first choice (best guess) treatment, which may be modified as a result of laboratory identification of organisms from pus, blood cultures or elsewhere. This is:

Penicillin 1200 mg 6-hourly
Netilmicin 80 mg 8-hourly
Metronidazole 400 mg 6-hourly

The blood netilmicin level must be monitored daily to reduce the risk of toxicity, particularly if the patient's renal function is impaired, and a special regimen of treatment must be drawn up for the anuric patient. If the patient is already in established renal failure, cefuroxime is given instead of the penicillin/aminoglycoside combination.

Before antibiotics are used, specimens must be taken from every conceivable source, which obviously includes blood cultures, in an attempt to identify the cause of the illness. The dose of netilmicin recommended may be found not to produce adequate blood levels, and it should be constantly reviewed.

If this type of regimen does not bring about an improvement within 2 days the surgeons should be asked to consider re-exploration. If, in spite of the satisfactory drainage of an intra-abdominal abscess, the patient's condition is not improving, an additional infection site may be present and should be looked for.

Antibiotic regimens should not be changed until at least 5 days' treatment have been given, unless bacteriological evidence suggests the 'best guess' regime is completely wrong. No course of antibiotics should be continued for more than 7 days unless the patient has a source of infection which cannot be found or relieved. However, it cannot be overemphasized that the essential part of treatment is to discover the source of the infection, drain it or remove it.

Other aids to treatment of haemorrhagic shock

The space blanket

This is a lightweight aluminized sheet which is widely used by campers and climbers as a substitute for conventional bedding. Apart from its light weight there is some doubt as to the additional benefit this material has for the adventurous since it has been shown to have no better thermal qualities than the standard blanket, but in hospital it is used to wrap patients who are hypothermic as a result of trauma (with or without exposure) or surgical procedures. This subject is dealt with more comprehensively in Chapter 9. It has become standard practice to wrap a 'space blanket' around any patient who shows signs of peripheral or central cooling. If the patient's core temperature rises and his skin temperature remains static, the space blanket should be removed since the core temperature may overshoot and other treatment, which includes the use of chlorpromazine or alpha-adrenergic blockers, may be indicated. Physical methods or warming should not be used as a substitute for volume replacement or the use of alpha blocking agents.

The G-suit

This is an inflatable double-layered plastic bag which is wrapped around the patient in order to apply external counterpressure. Several sizes are available and they should envelop the patient from the nipple line to the ankles. It is inflated to 30 cm water pressure and is used to arrest retroperitoneal or intramuscular bleeding such as may occur from pelvic, lumbar or closed lower limb injuries. It is most frequently used for the pre- and post-operative care of patients with leaking abdominal aortic aneurysms and it can be effectively used to aid the safe transport of injured patients. (It has no place in the treatment of intra-abdominal, as distinct from retroperitoneal, bleeding.) It may be applied for periods in excess of 24 hours, and although when it is properly used it does not interfere with spontaneous ventilation, most patients who require this form of treatment can benefit from controlled ventilation.

The G-suit can easily cause skin necrosis and it must be carefully applied, with particular attention being paid to contact points between the knees and ankles, which should be separated by sponge pads.

The MAST suit is a similar device which may have some advantages. The lower limbs of the suit are separated, which allows it to be used as a splint during transportation.

References

Cowley, R.A. & Trump, B. (1982) *Pathophysiology of Shock, Anoxia and Ischemia.* 710 pp. Baltimore and London: Williams and Wilkins.

Flear, C.T.G. & Singh, C.M. (1973) Hyponatraemia and sick cells. *British Journal of Anaesthesia,* **45,** 976–983.

Hardaway, R. (1980) Treatment of severe shock with phenoxybenzamine. *Surgery, Gynecology and Obstetrics,* **151,** 725–734.

Jones, P. & Stoddart, J.C. (1977) Coagulation disorders. In *Recent Advances in Intensive Therapy 1* (Ed.) Ledingham I.McA. pp. 91–105. Edinburgh, London, New York: Churchill Livingstone.

Kerr, D.N.S. & Elliott, R.W. (1974) The pathogenesis of acute renal failure. In *Acute Renal Failure* (Ed.) Flynn C.T. pp. 9–36. Lancaster: Mediçal and Technical Publishing Co.

Kreger, B.E., Craven D.E. & McCabe, W.R. (1980) Gram-negative bacteremia; re-evaluation of clinical features and treatment in 612 patients. *American Journal of Medicine,* **68,** 344–355.

Rosenbaum, R.W., Hayes, M.F., Marello, D.C. & Matsumoto, T. (1973) The importance of pulmonary artery pressure monitoring. *Surgery, Gynecology, Obstetrics,* **136,** 1–4.

Rudowski, W. & Kostrzewska, E. (1976) Blood substitutes. *Annals of the Royal College of Surgeons of England,* **58,** 115–125.

Stein, L., Berand, J.J., Morisette, M. et al. (1975) Pulmonary edema during volume infusion. *Circulation,* **52,** 483–489.

Stoddart, J.C. (1976) Fluid balance and acute cardiovascular failure. In *Recent Advances in Anaesthesia and Analgesia 12* (Ed.) Langton Hewer, C. & Atkinson, R.J., pp. 174–198. Edinburgh, London, New York: Churchill Livingstone.

Stoddart, J.C. (1982) Hospital acquired infection. In *Care of the Critically Ill Patient.* (Ed.) Tinker, J. and Rapin, M. Chapter 52. Berlin, New York: Springer Verlag.

Tinker, J. (1979) A pharmacological approach to the treatment of shock. *British Journal of Hospital Medicine*, **21** (3), 13–18.

Wallace, J. (1977) *Blood Transfusion for Clinicians*. 320 pp. Edinburgh, London, New York: Churchill Livingstone.

Wilson, R.F., Sibbald, W.J. & Jaanimagi, J.L. (1976) Haemodynamic effects of dopamine in critically ill septic patients. *Journal of Surgical Research*, **20** (3), 163–172.

3

Trauma and the Upper Airway

From the moment his training in the specialty begins, the anaesthetist is made aware of the importance of maintaining the patency of the upper airway. All too many of the deaths associated with anaesthesia are due to asphyxia, and this is also a common cause of death after trauma. Many individual factors are involved, but the ultimate cause is either (1) asphyxia due to coma, or (2) asphyxia due to obstruction or injury to the upper respiratory tract.

These conditions are not mutually exclusive. A patient whose level of consciousness is depressed may be unable to maintain his airway if it is partially obstructed by something which is only a minor nuisance to a conscious patient. In Chapter 1 it was stated that the assessment of respiratory function could be difficult in the absence of blood gas analysis. On the other hand, if asphyxia or respiratory depression are recognized quickly their treatment may be simple and have gratifying results. Upper and lower airway problems caused by burns are discussed in Chapter 7.

Asphyxia due to coma

There are many definitions of coma, but in this chapter it is defined as a level of consciousness which is inadequate for the patient's safety. General anaesthesia is controlled coma and the prevention or management of asphyxia due to coma should be second nature to the anaesthetist. The most difficult part of the exercise is recognition of the need for intervention. Patients who are apnoeic, or those who are cyanosed and breathing noisily, with blood bubbles or vomit issuing from the nose or mouth and using their accessory muscles of respiration present no diagnostic problem. However, the comatose patient cannot usually respond to hypoxia in this classic fashion and may slip quietly into irreversible hypoxic brain damage without obvious external signs. The difficulty of recognizing hypoxia in the field, or when the patient is cold, dirty or exsanguinated, has already been alluded to.

Every patient who is not fully conscious and talking is in danger of asphyxia. A patient who has sustained a head injury, no matter how trivial it may seem, should always be carefully watched. Any traumatized patient who has been given a narcotic analgesic by any route should be considered to be at risk since the absorption and effects of natural or synthetic narcotics are especially unpredictable in the shocked patient.

Any patient who is thought to be at risk should be placed under continuous observation until the outcome is clear. At its most basic, observation means engaging the patient in conversation at short intervals but it includes recording the rate, rhythm and depth of ventilation.

Aspiration pneumonia

Every comatose patient is also in danger from the inhalation of saliva, blood or gastric contents into the air passages. It is often stated that aspiration pneumonitis is a relatively rare condition, but nothing could be further from the truth. In fact, it is one of the commonest causes of death of patients who have undergone surgery under general anaesthesia, or who are even mildly obtunded by head injury or sedative drugs. Its association with upper airway injuries should need no emphasis.

The other misapprehension is that inhalation of foreign material is an obvious or even dramatic event, accompanied by vomiting, choking or cyanosis, whereas in many cases it is completely silent, and recognizable only after radiographic examination, blood gas analysis or autopsy examination. Only rarely does aspiration follow active vomiting; much more often it is the sequel to an unrecognized surge of gastric contents passing through a relaxed cardiac sphincter, bypassing a nasogastric tube and trickling unannounced down the patient's trachea.

Recognizing airway inadequacy

Every patient who is even moderately obtunded should be regarded as being in danger of airway obstruction, aspiration or respiratory depression. The approach to such a patient should be in the following sequence:

1 After pressure is applied to the chin to occlude the airway, does the patient react appropriately? (If not, pass to 4.)
2 Is he lying on his back and snoring? (If so, turn him on his side and pass to 3.)
3 Can the patient cough on request? (If not prepare to use a sucker and try 4.)
4 Will the patient allow a Guedel airway to be inserted? (If so, leave it in place and try 5.)
5 Will the patient tolerate laryngoscopy and pharyngeal suction? (If so, move to 6.)
6 Will the patient tolerate endotracheal intubation? (Go immediately to 7.)
7 Will the patient accept controlled ventilation? (If so, provide it.)

The author *always* uses the long-blade Macintosh laryngoscope for larger children and adults since this simplifies even the most difficult intubation and there is no additional difficulty with its use.

Even if the patient is making respiratory efforts, if he will allow the medical attendant to control his ventilation, IPPV must be applied and the cause of ventilatory depression looked for. A quick neurological examination along the lines described in Chapter 1 should be performed, with particular attention being paid to the pupils and ears (for bleeding from the external auditory canal). As soon as possible a neurologist or neurosurgeon should be asked to see the patient and drugs which may have a sedative, analgesic or neuro-muscular blocking effect must be withheld. This subject is discussed in greater detail in Chapter 8.

Asphyxia due to injury to the upper airway

Many patients who have suffered upper airway trauma die before help can be provided, but others can be saved with the minimum of equipment. Placing the patient in the lateral, head down position is frequently all that is required. An efficient suction device and a nasopharyngeal tube or Guedel airway may be life-saving. The nasopharyngeal airway is probably the most under-used device in anaesthesia and resuscitation, but it may transform the situation for a struggling asphyxiating patient and a desperate anaesthetist. Although specially designed nasopharyngeal tubes are available, any tube which will pass atraumatically through the nose into the oropharynx is equally satisfactory, so long as it is inserted for the correct distance. This is best determined by listening to the end of the tube. When the position is found to be satisfactory, a safety pin should be inserted from side-to-side through the tube, to prevent it from slipping further down. The pin should not be allowed to prevent the passage of a suction catheter.

Facio-maxillary injuries

The most common major facio-maxillary injury is a fracture of the mandible, with or without soft tissue damage. Mandibular fractures rarely cause airway difficulties although if treatment includes wiring the jaws together the patient may present an immediate post-anaesthetic problem and occasionally soft tissue damage with haematoma formation or oedema may obstruct the airway.

Most of the difficulties associated with trauma to the upper airways are minimized if surgery can be postponed for 24 hours or more after the injury. The bleeding which results from the injury may occasionally be extensive enough to require volume replacement. However, much of the blood which is lost is swallowed and may be regurgitated, and the combination of general anaesthesia, airway difficulties and a full stomach is unnecessarily dangerous. The indications for the immediate treatment of upper airway trauma include imminent asphyxia and, occasionally, major arterial or venous bleeding, particularly when these are caused by direct injury (penetrating wound, self-inflicted laceration). Cosmetic or convenience considerations must never be allowed to influence what is a sensible decision. Most facio-maxillary surgeons are prepared to wait for at least 24 hours after the injury before asking the anaesthetist for his assistance. By this time the bleeding will have stopped and the patient's stomach should have emptied itself. Nevertheless, as a precaution a nasogastric tube must be passed and the stomach emptied.

PRE-OPERATIVE ASSESSMENT

Unless there is a dire emergency, it should be possible to obtain some basic clinical and radiographic information before the patient is anaesthetized.

If the patient is conscious he should be asked to carry out a series of manoeuvres which are designed to obtain the following information:

1   Can he flex and extend his neck? (He must not be helped to do this.)

2 How far can he open his mouth?
3 Can he move his tongue freely?
4 Can he vocalize?
5 Does he develop stridor when coughing or breathing rapidly?
6 Can he breathe through one or both nostrils?
7 Has he any loose teeth, crowns, bridgework, bone fragments?

Radiographs should be taken of the face, soft tissues of the neck, chest and, where indicated, of the cervical spine. Occasionally, gross displacement of the larynx and trachea may be recognized. Foreign material originating in the mouth or stomach may already have been inhaled into the tracheobronchial tree and this should be noted before the patient is anaesthetized and a written record inserted in the notes.

Cervical cord injuries

Approximately 2% of patients who have sustained facio-maxillary trauma have some degree of cervical cord damage, although only a small number of these develop serious neurological injury. The cervical cord may be injured in a wide variety of vehicular and industrial accidents. In some cases the patient already has a neurological deficit by the time the anaesthetist is asked to see him. In others the bony injury may result in instability of his cervical spine which can be aggravated by any movement. If any doubt exists the opinion of an orthopaedic surgeon should be obtained, particularly if the patient is to undergo general anaesthesia with intubation.

Fortunately for the patient (and for the anaesthetist) in most cases extension is safer than flexion and laryngoscopy and endotracheal intubation should present no real problem. However, the patient must be moved as little and as gently as possible. The pre-operative assessment should include a full neurological examination so that any pre-existing damage can be noted, and not blamed upon the anaesthetist's ministrations.

Some orthopaedic surgeons elect to perform an immediate spinal fusion if the patient has a cervical cord injury, either by the anterior or posterior approach, and the patient may arrive in the anaesthetic room in a Stryker frame with skull traction already applied. Although the full stomach must be considered, anaesthesia with cricoid pressure and intubation are not usually a major problem. However, in at least one centre of excellence the patient is presented to the anaesthetist in the prone position and this has to be maintained during induction and intubation. Local expertise is of a high order and the technique is apparently not difficult to learn. Presumably it is learned quickly. Induction is with thiopentone followed by suxamethonium and the anaesthetist adopts the kneeling (prayer?) position for intubation. The patient's head and neck are fixed by an assistant who is very familiar with the technique.

It has been suggested that patients with cervical cord injury who have other injuries should not be given suxamethonium since on at least one occasion this has caused cardiac arrest due to hyperkalaemia. Although this must be a very uncommon event, the introduction of atracurium should have reduced the need for the use of suxamethonium. The patient's pre-anaesthetic serum potassium level should be measured as part of the routine pre-operative laboratory investigations.

Occasionally middle-aged or elderly patients who have suffered whiplash type injuries present with dense paralysis of the upper limbs and some degree of paresis of the legs. This results from hyperextension causing an ischaemic central cord lesion which is eminently recoverable. In this condition no further neck extension is permissible and intubation requires particular care.

The use of the fibre-optic bronchoscope

If the patient needs a general anaesthetic and the orthopaedic surgeon or radiologist suggests that the cervical cord injury is unstable, intubation may present special difficulties. It is in this situation that the fibre-optic broncho-scope is particularly useful. The fibre-optic laryngoscope may be used, although the absence of a suction channel, its limited depth of focus and its restricted mobility are sometimes a problem.

If a fibre-optic device is to be used, an attempt should first be made to stabilize the head and neck with a plastic collar or sandbags, although this is mainly for the patient's comfort and to remind the attendant of the dangers. The presence of soft tissue injuries may make this an impractical recommen-dation. The patient should then be given a full explanation of the manoeuvres the anaesthetist intends to perform. If he is in severe pain or very apprehensive, a small dose of an opiate (5 mg morphine) or a benzodiazepine such as 4 mg lorazepam or midazolam may be given intravenously. Then the upper airways, including both nostrils, are generously sprayed with 4% lignocaine.

If the patient can open his mouth, the pharynx, larynx and trachea are sprayed under direct vision. If not, this is done blindly using a flexible lignocaine spray introduced through the anaesthetized nostril. Additional topical anaesthesia can be obtained by injecting 2 ml 4% lignocaine through the cricothyroid membrane. This usually provokes coughing, but if not the patient should be asked to cough to distribute the local anaesthetic around the larynx and upper airway. At least three minutes should be allowed to elapse before the airway is approached. Then the fibre-optic bronchoscope is well lubricated and is threaded through the selected endotracheal tube so that at least 2.5 cm protrude beyond it. The tube has already been cut to the appropriate length and lubricated. The 'scope is then inserted through the nose and gently advanced into the oropharynx. If this provokes vigorous coughing it may be possible to inject more lignocaine down the suction channel of the 'scope from a 5 ml syringe. The dead-space of the suction channel is 2 ml. If the pharynx is full of blood or mucus, this should be aspirated. The 'scope is introduced into the trachea until it is below the vocal cords and the endotracheal tube can then be advanced over it. Anaesthesia is induced immediately afterwards and very few patients have any recollection of these manoeuvres.

Alternative methods of intubation

If a fibre-optic bronchoscope is not available, or if the patient is too small for the bronchoscope to be introduced, two other techniques may be used.

The first involves cricothyroid puncture. The patient is first given a small intravenous dose of lorazepam or midazolam and, after topical application of lignocaine to the mouth and pharynx, the skin over the cricothyroid membrane is anaesthetized with lignocaine and a Tuohy needle is introduced through the membrane into the trachea and further local anaesthesia instilled. The open tip of the needle is pointed towards the patient's head and an epidural catheter advanced through it. The patient can usually tell when the catheter enters his mouth, but if not it is visualized and the end drawn out with Magill forceps. If nasal intubation is essential, after the application of topical lignocaine a second catheter can be passed via a nostril into the mouth and the two ends tied or stitched together and the end of the transtracheal catheter withdrawn through the nostril. In either case the endotracheal tube is then threaded over the catheter while an assistant pulls on both ends to make it taut. The tube will then slide over the catheter into the trachea.

If neither of these methods succeeds, a tracheostomy should first be performed under local anaesthesia and the patient then anaesthetized. This is often regarded as a procedure of last resort, but anything is preferable to allowing a patient to asphyxiate for want of a reliably patent airway, or to be exposed to the risk of permanent neurological damage through movement of the unstable head and neck. If the surgeon elects to use the anterior approach to the cervical cord, pre-operative tracheostomy is not possible.

These maneouvres can be used in other situations in which laryngoscopy and intubation are difficult.

Soft tissue injuries

Although extensive soft tissue injuries are themselves painful, manipulations such as laryngoscopy appear to cause little additional discomfort if proper care is taken. For this reason, and because of its intrinsic safety, awake intubation without topical anaesthesia is practised by many anaesthetists. If the patient is very distressed or in pain from other injuries, minimal analgesia, such as morphine 5 mg intravenously for an adult may be given and pre-oxygenation may be advisable. The patient is then told what to expect and asked to breathe slowly and deeply. The laryngoscope is then gradually advanced over the tongue and the endotracheal tube inserted during inspiration. This is often surprisingly easy and the patient can then be anaesthetized safely.

Occasionally, although the patient can maintain a satisfactory airway, because of tissue distortion the larynx cannot be visualised fully or at all. In this case, a gum-elastic bougie or flexible stilette should be inserted through the endotracheal tube with approximately 2.5 cm protruding beyond its tip. The bougie is then directed blindly around the obstruction into the larynx, and the tube is railroaded down the bougie or stilette and the patient anaesthetized. This technique may be used to aid difficult intubation in the anaesthetized patient and a stilette should always be available before induction of anaesthesia is attempted.

Very occasionally it is necessary to use a rigid paediatric or suckling bronchoscope as an emergency airway for adults because of extensive soft tissue damage, bleeding and distortion of the upper air passages. After insertion the patient can be anaesthetized through the bronchoscope. Every anaesthetist should be adept with this instrument.

Under no circumstances should any form of intravenous induction agent or muscle relaxant be given to a patient if any doubt exists as to the patency of the airway or as to the ability of the anaesthetist to apply controlled ventilation by face-mask, should the patient become obstructed or apnoeic. If a patient who has suffered upper airway trauma has to be anaesthetized before an endotracheal tube can be inserted, only inhalational techniques should be used. Halothane/oxygen or enflurane/oxygen are the methods of choice.

POST-OPERATIVE CARE

Patients who have undergone extensive facio-maxillary surgery are almost equally in danger of asphyxia after the surgical procedure as during induction of anaesthesia. In some cases this is because of continued bleeding or oedema; in others, it is because the patient's maxilla and mandible have had to be stabilized in such a way that the patient cannot guarantee to protect his own airway (Figure 6). In these circumstances the nasopharyngeal airway is very useful. This should be inserted at the end of surgery so that it lies behind the

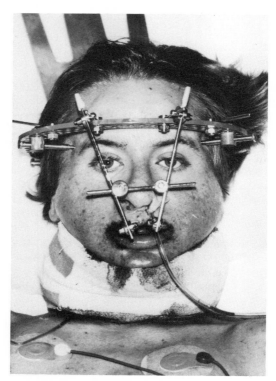

Figure 6. This patient underwent a surgical procedure to stabilize her jaw and the middle third of her face. She presented difficulties with both intubation and extubation.

tongue and guarantees that oedema cannot obstruct the oropharynx. Alternatively, when the patient is awake and breathing normally the cuffed nasotracheal tube which has been used for anaesthesia can be deflated and withdrawn from the trachea but allowed to remain in the oropharynx. In either case the tube is not removed until 2 to 24 hours after surgery is completed, when the patient is known to be able to maintain his own airway. This can be established by occluding the end of the tube and ensuring that he can still breathe freely.

Nasopharyngeal tubes can be used to facilitate aspiration of blood or mucus from the pharynx. If an absorbent pack is placed in the oropharynx by the anaesthetist or surgeon, this must be removed before the tube is withdrawn.

DIRECT TRACHEAL INJURY

Occasionally the larynx or trachea is injured by external violence; two similar types of accident may cause tracheal compression which is either quickly fatal or may present difficulties when the patient reaches hospital. Children riding tricycles (or bicycles) and adults riding motor cycles frequently have their forward progress abruptly arrested, and occasionally the rider falls forward over the handlebars and strikes his neck on the stem. A similar injury is produced by a child's swing coming back and striking him in the neck. In either case the symptoms include acute distress with cyanosis, dyspnoea and stridor and blood-stained sputum bubbling from the mouth. Whenever possible, before attempting to insert any airway of any sort the patient should be given an inhalational anaesthetic of halothane in oxygen, exactly as if he had epiglottitis or laryngotracheitis. If the patient settles with this treatment the emergency is over and the next step can be carefully considered. However, in many cases an attempt has to be made to insert an artificial airway. Standard endotracheal tubes may be too soft for this purpose and the most effective airway is the rigid bronchoscope. This must be inserted as gently as possible, and the smallest size chosen which will provide an effective airway. Even an adult can be adequately oxygenated through a suckling broncho-scope with the aid of the Sanders injector (Figure 7). Carbon dioxide accumulation is of no importance in this type of emergency. Once the obstruction has been bypassed, the situation should be allowed to stabilize and the injury explored under anaesthesia, and a tracheostomy performed if necessary. Some form of continuous intravenous technique should be used, such as ketamine or the etomidate/fentanyl sequence. Most tracheal injuries due to trauma involve the thyroid cartilage and upper tracheal rings. The surgeon who carries out the exploration must decide whether or not to make the stoma through the damaged area. This is probably the site of choice since the traumatized trachea may become stenosed, and it is better not to create an additional area of potential stenosis by fashioning a tracheostomy below this. In addition, if the stoma is made below the third tracheal ring, it may be difficult to prevent the tip of the tracheostomy tube entering the right main bronchus.

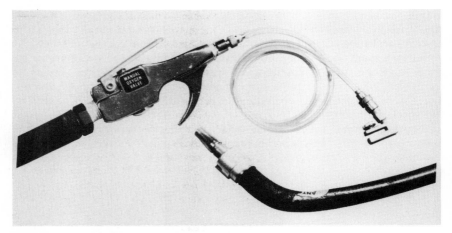

Figure 7. The Sanders injector. This device can be used during bronchoscopy and also as a means of applying controlled ventilation in difficult situations.

Penetrating wounds

The cervical part of the trachea is sometimes opened by direct stab wounds and similar incidents. The resulting haemorrhage may be life-threatening, but airway obstruction may also present a problem. Frequently the most effective treatment is to intubate the patient's trachea through the laceration. Oxygenation, anaesthesia and surgery can then be achieved safely.

Of all the types of upper airway trauma encountered, blunt tracheal injury is the only one in which immediate formal tracheostomy is the treatment of choice, once the airway has been controlled.

Burns and scalds

The larynx and trachea may also be damaged by burns, scalds or hot gases. Usually the vocal cords go into spasm when presented with hot material and most injuries are restricted to the supraglottic area. However, occasionally inflammable gases ignite after inhalation, and patients may survive after having inhaled flame or superheated steam since the thermal capacity of the lower airways is considerable. In this circumstance the anaesthetist must simply do what he can to provide an airway and oxygenation. Endotracheal intubation may be possible, or the bronchoscope may be utilized. If the supraglottic area is extensively damaged, tracheal insufflation or the crico-thyrotomy cannula (Figure 9) may buy time for an elective tracheostomy to be performed. Exceptionally, an emergency tracheostomy without benefit of oxygenation or any form of anaesthesia may be the last resort, although in the author's experience it is rarely life-saving.

If the injury is restricted to the upper airway, the patient can be allowed to breathe spontaneously through the endotracheal or tracheostomy tube. The management thereafter is a matter for trial and error, but usually the patient's upper airway is examined under general anaesthesia on the third day after intubation and the subsequent course decided by the findings. Children with scalds to the upper airway can usually be extubated within seven days of the incident. Although corticosteroids are often given in this situation, they confer no benefit and may increase the hazard of local and secondary infection.

The bronchoscope used as an airway

The use of the rigid bronchoscope as an artificial airway and for applying controlled ventilation has been mentioned in the preceding sections. When combined with the Sanders injector it can be life-saving but, unless a prior modification has been made to the injector, the patient has to be ventilated with oxygen which is diluted with entrained air. Most anaesthetic departments can adapt the injector so that it can be used with Entonox cylinders, and this is useful if a surgical procedure such as a tracheostomy has to be performed although the level of analgesia is unpredictable. An intravenous agent such as ketamine or the fentanyl/etomidate sequence can be used while the patient is being ventilated through the bronchoscope.

ACTION FOR THE DIRE EMERGENCY

Rarely, a patient may arrive in the hospital with such extensive damage to the upper airways that he is virtually unable to breathe and in imminent danger of death. Rather more frequently, patients who have been in the hospital for a short time develop rapidly progressive airway obstruction due to further bleeding or oedema with tissue distortion. Exceptionally, children with laryngotracheitis or epiglottitis may present the same desperate picture, although orotracheal intubation under halothane/oxygen anaesthesia is usually possible. In these circumstances there are three possible forms of treatment.

Emergency tracheostomy

The results of emergency tracheostomy without any prior oxygenation or local or general anaesthesia are uniformly bad, usually because the person on the spot has never done one before, but also because upper airway obstruction is always accompanied by venous engorgement which causes massive haemorrhage, and because of violent and uncontrollable movements on the part of the patient. A good argument can be made out for teaching all medical personnel how to perform a tracheostomy, but this is so rarely needed that the opportunities for teaching are exceptional and the recommendation impractical.

Transtracheal insufflation

This is a relatively simple procedure. A 'nick' is made in the skin over the cricothyroid membrane with a pointed scalpel blade and a large diameter (14 gauge or larger) intravenous cannula is pushed into the trachea and directed caudally. After the metal inner cannula has been removed, pure oxygen can be

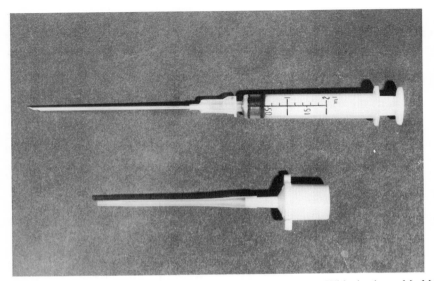

Figure 8. How an intravenous cannula may be used as an airway. (With thanks to Mr M. Clyburn, SRN.)

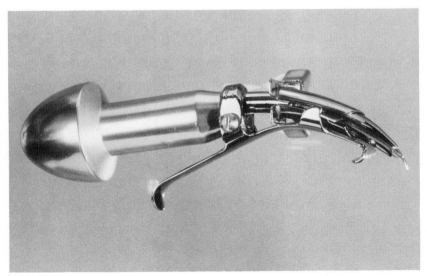

Figure 9. The Penlon cricothyrotomy cannula. For a full description see text.

blown down the cannula in sufficient volume to maintain life. The Sanders injector can be attached directly to the hub of the cannula and the patient inflated with oxygen. Alternatively, the standard 15 mm taper, size 3.5 mm endotracheal tube connector can be fitted into any luer-fitting cannula and then attached to an oxygen source or anaesthetic machine outlet (Figure 8). The author has experience of this technique being used to oxygenate and anaesthetize a two-year-old child while a formal, successful tracheostomy was performed. Alternatively, the attendant can simply blow through the intratracheal cannula and provide enough oxygenation for a child. Expiration presents no problem.

Commercial devices which are intended to be used as described above are available but have no advantages over the improvised methods.

Emergency cricothyrotomy

The Penlon cricothyrotomy cannula is a device which is designed to relieve upper airway obstruction (Figure 9). The patient's head is extended and a horizontal skin incision 0.5 cm long is made over the cricothyroid membrane. This is said not to be essential, but it probably makes the procedure easier. The cannula blade is then pushed through the intervening tissues until the trachea is entered. The blade is retracted and the integral metal dilators pushed forward over the blade into the trachea, opened, and a cuffed size 4 tracheostomy tube inserted through the dilators. This instrument cannot be used for children under the age of 4 years. If the kit is not available, a cricothyrotomy can be performed by standard means. This is much safer than an emergency tracheostomy but is still a hazardous procedure.

References

Cloward, R.B. (1980) Acute cervical cord injuries. *Clinical Symposia*, **32** (1), 2–32.

Fraser, A. & Edmonds Seal, J. (1982) Spinal cord injuries. A review of the problems facing the anaesthetist. *Anaesthesia*, **37** (11), 1084–1098.

Jacoby, J.J., Hamelbeg, W., Ziegler, C.H. et al (1956) Transtracheal resuscitation. *Journal of the American Medical Association*, **162**, 625–628.

Klain, M., Keszler, H. & Brader, E. (1981) High frequency jet ventilation in cardio-pulmonary resuscitation. *Critical Care Medicine*, **9**, 421–422.

Messeter, K.H. & Pettersen, K.I. (1980) Endotracheal intubation with the fibre-optic broncho-scope. *Anaesthesia*, **35** (3), 294–298.

Sanders, R.D. (1967) Two ventilating attachments for bronchoscopes. *Delaware Medical Journal*, **39**, 170–174.

Snow, J.C., Kripke, B.J., Session, G.P. & Fink A.J. (1973) Cardiovascular collapse following succinylcholine in a paraplegic patient. *Paraplegia*, **11**, 199–200.

4

The Management of Chest Injuries

Most major chest injuries result from road traffic accidents, with a small number being caused by other types of trauma. In hospital, an occasional patient may be seen whose chest injuries have been produced by closed chest cardiac massage. Rarely, patients who have undergone extensive thoracic or thoraco-abdominal surgery may present a similar problem. In all of these situations the initial management is the same. This is based upon the immediate effects of the injury and concentrates upon: (1) cardiocirculatory resuscitation; (2) pain relief; and (3) gas exchange. The order of priorities is discussed in Chapter 1.

Cardiocirculatory resuscitation

Resuscitation is discussed in Chapter 2 but it should be realized that patients who have sustained major chest injuries may exsanguinate with no external evidence of blood loss. One half of the thoracic cavity can easily accommodate the entire blood volume. Fractured ribs often tear intercostal or internal mammary arteries, and the lungs are very vascular and frequently bleed profusely. More dramatic bleeding may result from damage to the aorta, the vena cava or the heart.

Many patients with chest injuries also have injuries elsewhere which result in significant blood loss and for which the optimum treatment includes large volume fluid replacement. The need to maintain perfusion and at the same time protect the lungs from the danger of overtransfusion creates a conflict in the treatment of patients with multiple injuries. This explains in part why patients who also have other injuries require more prolonged supportive treatment than those whose injuries are localized to the thorax and its contents. All lung injuries are accompanied by the accumulation of fluid in the pulmonary interstitium or in the alveoli, for which the treatment includes fluid restriction and the use of diuretics. A compromise must be found between the needs for volume replacement and for fluid restriction. As soon as the acute phase of resuscitation is completed, and provided that there is no evidence of continued blood loss, the fluid intake must be restricted to not more than 1 litre for the next 24 hours. If the patient has suffered extensive pulmonary contusions and is hypoxic, he should be given frusemide 40 mg intravenously 12-hourly. This regimen should be continued for up to 3 days, or until the blood urea starts to rise. If no sustained improvement in the radiographic appearance or blood gas exchange has been achieved at the end of this period, the frusemide should be discontinued but thereafter fluid overload should be avoided at all costs. If the patient is oliguric or in frank renal failure from the time of admission, early haemodialysis must be considered.

It is more important to protect damaged lungs from the ill effects of overtransfusion than to protect the kidneys from hypovolaemia. There is little doubt that the mortality rate from acute renal failure is lower than that from acute post-traumatic respiratory failure.

Pain relief

Even the most trivial chest wall injury is painful, and the patient may also be in pain from other injuries. Pain restricts respiratory movements and interferes with the efficiency of coughing and of expectoration. If the patient will not or cannot cough, he is in danger of atelectasis, and the ability to expectorate is one of the most useful guides to the severity of the injury. Pain also greatly increases tissue oxygen consumption. The patient must therefore be given effective pain relief as soon as possible, but whichever method is used its side-effects must constantly be borne in mind. Relief of pain may enable the patient to breathe more deeply and to cough and expectorate. On the other hand it may also cause his respiratory centre to ignore the effects of hypoxia and hypercapnia and encourage the retention of secretions (page 64).

Problems of gas exchange

Paradoxical ventilation

Chest trauma interferes with gas exchange through the mechanisms referred to above but, more obviously, chest wall instability restricts respiratory movements and may cause paradoxical ventilation. This is defined as a condition in which the movement of part of the thoracic cage (and/or diaphragm) is in the opposite direction to the phase of ventilation. It is caused either by fractures in two places in the same rib or ribs, or the combination of rib fractures with costochondral fracture-dislocation. If the sternum is also fractured, a further cause for instability is created.

Paradoxical ventilation may be of a minor degree, affecting only one segment of the chest wall, or it may be so extensive that no effective alveolar ventilation or gas exchange can take place. If one side of the chest is totally unstable it is theoretically possible for the respiratory movements to move gas from one lung to the other—the so-called pendelluft (pendulum breathing)— without any external gas exchange taking place. Unless this is treated rapidly it is incompatible with life.

In recent years the effects of small areas of paradoxical ventilation have been shown to be of little significance, although major chest wall instability always causes hypoxia and hypercapnia. On the other hand if the patient is given effective pain relief he is often able to ventilate adequately even in the presence of quite extensive bone injury, with or without paradox.

Penetrating injuries

Penetrating injuries and direct pulmonary trauma create problems which may demand urgent treatment such as the insertion of a chest drain or the use of an occlusive pack.

Pneumothorax, with or without haemothorax, is treated by intercostal drainage, the details of which are discussed on page 82. If the wound is obviously contaminated it is usual for prophylactic antibiotics to be given, although their value is debatable.

Penetrating wounds of the pericardium or heart with or without tamponade require urgent surgical treatment. The treatment of tamponade caused by closed trauma is described on page 80. If the aorta or vena cava is injured, prolonged emergency surgery with extensive blood loss is to be anticipated.

The lungs and bronchi are often damaged by penetrating wounds. Lobectomy or, rarely, pneumonectomy may be required.

Extensive intrathoracic haemorrhage and the need for urgent surgery present the anaesthetist with major problems. However, the overall management of this type of injury is not different from that of any patient who has to undergo intrathoracic surgery when inadequately prepared.

Pulmonary contusions

Small children who have suffered severe injury may have no obvious fractures but become hypoxic because of underlying pulmonary contusions. In other cases, although the bony injuries may be the most obvious result of chest trauma, the underlying pulmonary damage is usually of much greater importance. Pulmonary contusions create a true shunt because the blood-suffused alveoli interfere with gas exchange, resulting in hypoxia with an increased alveolar-to-arterial oxygen tension gradient. In addition, contused lung tissue readily becomes infected.

Patients with chest injuries usually underventilate because of pain and reduced mechanical efficiency. Underventilation always results in hypercapnia and, unless the patient is receiving oxygen-enriched air, hypoxia.

THE CLASSIFICATION OF THE SEVERITY OF CHEST INJURIES

This is based upon the patient's pre-incident physical status, the extent of chest trauma and any associated injuries.

The extent and result of the pulmonary injury

Some patients have such extensive pulmonary injury that with the methods of treatment currently available they cannot be expected to survive owing to the combined effects of hypoxia and intrathoracic bleeding. The initial assessment of the severity of the injury must include chest radiography and blood gas analysis, although it may be obvious at first sight and without the aid of these investigations that the patient requires oxygen therapy or ventilatory assistance. If the extent of the injury is not immediately apparent the patient must be kept under constant skilled observation and re-examined at intervals which are dictated by his overall physical status.

Blood gas analysis

Blood gas analysis may need to be repeated hourly until a firm decision can be made as to the extent of the injuries and the course of treatment required. Blood gas analysis must be performed after the patient has been given his first effective dose of an analgesic drug, particularly if he is somnolent or asleep, to exclude the possibility of respiratory depression.

The blood gas analysis results must be clearly charted since they are the only reliable indication of the progression of the lesion. During the first 48 hours after the injury, hypoxia without hypercapnia is usually due to pulmonary contusion, pneumothorax or pulmonary oedema. Arterial hypercapnia always means that the patient is underventilating either because of the injury(s) or its treatment. The causes include the use of narcotic analgesics or previously undiagnosed head injury, but in every case the attendant must be prepared to apply controlled ventilation. Ventilatory depression due to narcotics can be reversed with naloxone. At this stage in treatment only those drugs which can be easily reversed should be given. This excludes benzodiazepines.

If an injured patient becomes confused or begins to behave in a bizarre fashion, hypoxia is the most likely cause and the appropriate steps must be taken to identify and treat it. Brain damage (extradural and shearing injury) and fat embolism must also be included in the differential diagnosis. Sepsis is a common cause of post-traumatic confusion, but this complication usually develops later. Confusion is not a diagnosis but a symptom and confused patients must *never* be given sedative, narcotic or similar drugs until the cause of the symptom has been determined.

Chest radiography

Chest radiography is an essential part of the immediate and continuing assessment of chest trauma. In the first instance it will reveal the extent of the bone damage and of the underlying pulmonary contusions or other injury, although if only portable films can be taken, injuries to the sternum and anterior ribs will not be demonstrated and the shape and size of the heart cannot be determined accurately. It is quite common for previously unrecognized rib fractures to be identified days later during the course of treatment. Pulmonary contusions may not be apparent radiographically until up to 24 hours after the incident for reasons which are not obvious but may include the redistribution of tranfused fluids into the lung.

Whenever possible the films should be taken with the patient in the erect position. Erect films allow the size of the apical veins to be more accurately assessed and facilitate the recognition and quantification of pleural fluid; the position of the diaphragm and the presence of subphrenic gas may also be more readily determined.

Good quality lateral chest radiographs cannot be obtained after the patient is admitted to the intensive therapy unit or ward and, if possible, they should be taken in the x-ray department before admission.

After the treatment regimen has been decided upon, chest radiographs must be taken daily, or even more frequently. Complications which may arise during the course of treatment include new or recurrent pneumothorax or the appearance of delayed signs of aortic, pericardial or pleural bleeding. Evidence of bronchopneumonia or pulmonary oedema may also emerge.

Pre-existing health status

A patient who is suffering from an intercurrent disease at the time of his injury is at greater risk than a previously healthy person. These include cardiorespiratory disturbances such as hypertension, myocardial ischaemia and chronic obstructive airways disease, but musculo-skeletal disorders such as rheumatoid arthritis may also adversely influence the outcome of chest trauma. One of the commoner conditions which may have a profound bearing upon the prognosis is obesity, since this influences not only the consequences of the respiratory injury but the ease with which medical, surgical and nursing procedures can be carried out (Figure 10).

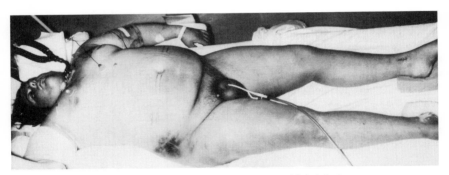

Figure 10. The influence of obesity on multiple injuries.

The effects of age

Major chest wall injuries are uncommon in small children both because of their epidemiology and because the infant and child has a thoracic cage which is almost infinitely malleable. Pulmonary contusions are also usually less severe and secondary infection a relatively minor problem. On the other hand elderly patients have very brittle bones which fracture readily, do not heal quickly and often pierce underlying structures. They are also more likely to suffer from intercurrent disease and have poor defence against traumatic insults and infection. Therefore their prognosis is proportionally worse than that of a younger person with injuries of the same extent.

Co-existing injury

Patients who suffer chest injuries following road traffic accidents frequently sustain extrathoracic injuries. Those which increase the morbidity of the chest injury include facio-maxillary, intra-abdominal and intracranial injuries.

Facio-maxillary injuries

Facio-maxillary injuries may cause airway obstruction, interfere with swallowing, expectoration and oral nutrition. If a patient requires facio-maxillary surgery, including interdental banding, the risk of major respiratory difficulties is greatly increased. This type of injury is also frequently associated with post-concussional confusion.

Intra-abdominal and pelvic injuries

If the patient has sustained intra-abdominal injuries which necessitate an abdominal exploratory laparotomy, the combination of pain and paralytic ileus interferes with respiratory movements and, in particular, prevents the patient from breathing deeply, coughing and expectorating.

Injuries which involve the lumbar vertebrae or pelvis always cause extensive retroperitoneal bleeding which has a similar effect. A perforated viscus or bowel resection presents an important potential source of infection, and the combination of intra-abdominal sepsis with thoracic trauma has a very high mortality rate.

These conditions may make oral or tube feeding impossible for a variable period. Since for the traumatized patient the maintenance of adequate nutrition is vital, parenteral feeding methods must be adopted, with the small but measurable increase in morbidity which inevitably follows.

Injuries which restrict the patient's ability to move in bed, either because of pain or extensive orthopaedic intervention, increase the risk of atelectasis, bronchopneumonia and pulmonary embolism. All patients with bony injuries (rarely, those with soft tissue injuries) are at risk of fat embolism (Chapter 6) and the potentially harmful effects of massive fluid replacement must be taken into account.

Level of consciousness

Any patient whose level of consciousness is impaired—because of direct brain damage, fat embolism or drugs—is in danger of pulmonary complications, either through his inability to co-operate with the nurses and physiotherapists, or because of respiratory depression and reduced airway protection. These factors weigh heavily in the balanced assessment of the severity of chest injuries. The relief of pain was referred to earlier, but patients who need systemic analgesics for long periods present a special problem.

Diaphragmatic rupture

This injury is relatively rare and is usually caused by trauma to the anterior abdominal wall, although the association between acetabular fractures and diaphragmatic rupture has been recognized for many years. The force is transmitted from the hip joint through the abdominal vicera and part or all of the stomach, small or large bowel and, occasionally, the spleen herniate into the thoracic cavity. Although injuries to the left hemidiaphragm are more frequently recognized, autopsy examination indicates that the right hemidiaphragm may also be injured, but it retains its normal outline because of the position of the liver.

The diagnosis of diaphragmatic rupture may be suggested by the clinical presentation. Dyspnoea and abdominal paradoxical ventilation may be suggestive, and the radiographic appearance may provide confirmatory evidence. The left hemidiaphragm may obviously be distorted and a visceral gas shadow may be visible in the left thoracic cavity. The diagnosis can be confirmed by passing a radio-opaque nasogastric tube; if the stomach has herniated, the position of the tube will make this obvious. If barium is injected down the nasogastric tube, the stomach or other hollow viscus may be seen to be above the diaphragm.

Occasionally the diagnosis is not made until many years after the event since the symptoms and signs may be innocuous. It may be an incidental finding, or the patient may complain of slowly increasing dyspnoea. Heartburn may also be a problem. Even complete diaphragmatic rupture with herniation of the spleen, stomach and other viscera may give rise to no complaints.

If the injury causes symptoms, which may include small bowel obstruction, surgical treatment may be required, but if possible surgical intervention should be delayed until the patient has recovered from his other injuries.

Bronchial injuries

The lower trachea and major bronchi are well protected from the effects of external chest trauma, and the type of injury which is violent enough to cause damage to these structures usually causes death very quickly because of damage to other structures.

Patients who survive are usually shocked, hypoxic and dyspnoeic and produce blood-stained sputum. They may have surgical emphysema which is localized to the supraclavicular region and base of the neck and have blood bubbles issuing from the mouth and nose. Chest radiography usually shows complete atelectasis of the affected lung together with mediastinal emphysema, but the cause can be confirmed only by bronchoscopy. The bronchus is usually found to be torn approximately 2 cm from the carina, causing complete obstruction of the distal segment. This condition is treated surgically and the results are usually good. As with many of the injuries described in this chapter, the diagnosis may occasionally be unrecognized until many months later. The results of delayed surgery are also said to be very good with full recovery of respiratory function.

THE TREATMENT OF CHEST INJURIES

After taking the above factors into consideration the severity of chest injuries can be tabulated as shown in Figure 11. This demonstrates the cumulative deleterious effects of factors which include increasing age, coma and intra-abdominal injuries. Although it is not intended to be fully comprehensive or to be applied rigidly, the classification is the principal guide to the regimen of treatment which the patient requires.

GRADE 1	GRADE 2	GRADE 3
Young patient Multiple ribs Nil else	Grade 1 + Ileus Hypoxic	Grade 2 + Obtunded
Middle aged Fit Few ribs	Middle aged Bronchitic Few ribs Hypoxic	Grade 2 + Ileus
	Elderly Few ribs Frail	Grade 2 + Hypoxic

Figure 11. A guide to the assessment of the severity of chest injuries.

Patients who have sustained grade 1 injuries require:
1 Titrated analgesia
2 Physiotherapy
3 Mobilization

Patients with grade 2 injuries require:
1 Titrated analgesia
2 Physiotherapy
3 Tracheostomy
4 Spontaneous ventilation with oxygen enrichment

Patients with grade 3 injuries require:
1 Titrated analgesia
2 Physiotherapy
3 Tracheostomy
4 Controlled ventilation with oxygen enrichment

This assessment must be repeated at frequent short intervals until the patient's condition stabilizes, since unexpected deterioration may occur. This implies that he should be observed in an intensive therapy unit.

Patients who require positive pressure ventilation usually have extensive pulmonary contusions and a wide Aa gradient. However, provided that the contused lung does not become grossly infected and that overtransfusion is avoided, most patients with grade 3 injuries should be able to breathe spontaneously through a tracheostomy after five to seven days of controlled ventilation. Occasionally this period has to be extended to two to three weeks. The mortality rate from chest injuries after the first 48 hours is largely dictated by the presence or absence of intra-abdominal and pulmonary infection.

The analgesia problem

The importance of pain relief was emphasized at the beginning of this chapter, but it was pointed out that sedation and analgesia could have undesirable side-effects which include respiratory depression and lack of patient co-operation. If the patient has suffered grade 1 injuries almost any analgesic drug can be used so long as its effects are monitored, but as soon as he obtains maximal pain relief he must be encouraged to move around freely if his other injuries present no obstacle. He must be taught the importance of deep breathing and expectoration, and his sputum carton must be examined frequently to ensure he is carrying out his instructions.

For many years tight adhesive strapping was applied over rib fractures to reduce respiratory movement and thus to relieve pain. Unfortunately, although this undoubtedly gives some pain relief it also increases the likelihood of atelectasis in the underlying area of the lung, and this form of treatment has a very limited place—as, for example, at half-time on the rugby field.

For patients with grade 1 or 2 injuries there is no doubt at all that the ideal form of pain relief is achieved with continuous thoracic epidural analgesia, and for many patients with grade 2 injuries effective analgesia obviates the need for tracheostomy. The case report which follows demonstrates this point.

Figure 12 shows the chest radiographs of a 40-year-old patient who was involved in a road traffic accident after a drinking bout. He had double fractures of ribs three to ten inclusive on the left side and he was obese, had a history of chronic obstructive airways disease due to cigarette smoking, was an alcoholic and also had a fractured femoral shaft. He had a large area of paradoxical ventilation, and within 12 hours of sustaining the injury he showed radiographic evidence of extensive pulmonary contusions and atelectasis, with a greatly reduced arterial oxygen tension (Figure 12b). An epidural catheter was inserted at the T4/5 interspace and 8 ml of 0.5% bupivacaine injected. Within 20 minutes complete relief of chest pain was achieved and the patient was able to breathe deeply, cough and expectorate. The pain relief also appeared to reduce the severity of paradoxical chest movements and 12 hours later there was almost total resolution of the clinical and radiographic signs of atelectasis (Figure 12c). Epidural analgesia was maintained for four days, at the end of which the patient was able to breathe freely with only minimal pain.

It was considered inadvisable to extend the epidural analgesia to relieve the pain from his fractured femur, and for this the patient was given buprenorphine 0.4 mg intramuscularly eight hourly. Buprenorphine rarely causes respiratory depression although, like most powerful analgesics, it may cause nausea, vomiting and vertigo.

Occasionally epidural analgesia may not be entirely satisfactory, either because the block is patchy or because so many thoracic segments need to be blocked that the patient becomes hypotensive. A patchy block may be corrected by withdrawing the catheter slightly, but it may have to be supplemented with systemic analgesics such as buprenorphine. If the patient has suffered very extensive chest injuries which cannot be adequately treated

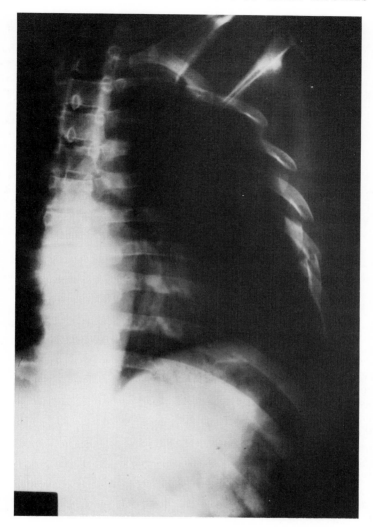

Figure 12a. The chest radiograph of a 40-year-old patient involved in a road traffic accident. An oblique film showing the fractures in ribs 2–10.

by epidural analgesia it may be advisable to downgrade the classification and treat him accordingly.

Tachyphylaxis may be another problem, although in the author's experience it is very uncommon and usually due to catheter displacement.

When the top-up dose has been determined, analgesia should be maintained with a syringe pump. If the patient has no other injuries and a clockwork or battery-powered syringe pump is available, he should be encouraged to walk around the ward.

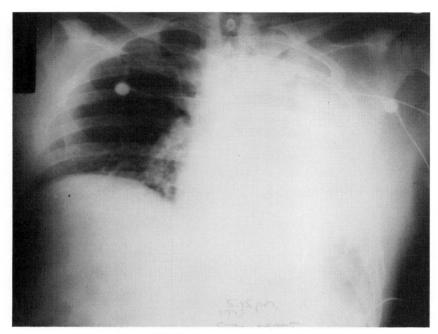

Figure 12b. The same patient 24 hours later.

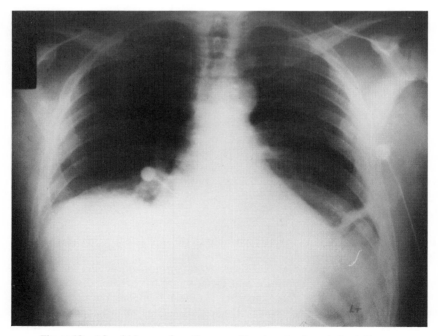

Figure 12c. After 24 hours of continuous epidural analgesia and physiotherapy.

In the uncomplicated case it is usually possible to dispense with epidural analgesia after four to five days. Patients who have persistent severe chest pain on coughing or while receiving physiotherapy can be given extra pain relief with Entonox, or small doses of systemic narcotics.

Endotracheal intubation and tracheostomy care

In addition to adequate pain relief, patients with grade 2/3 injuries usually require a tracheostomy. Its function is:
1 To permit the efficient aspiration of secretions and blood.
2 To facilitate the more efficient application of oxygen therapy and humidification.
3 To allow the nurse to measure and record the patient's tidal volume and minute volume.
4 To allow controlled ventilation to be applied.

Although a tracheostomy also reduces the anatomical dead space by 50–70 ml, this is of little additional benefit for the traumatized patient.
    Occasionally it may be possible to postpone or avoid the need for a tracheostomy by passing an endotracheal tube, particularly if the clinical presentation suggests that the incident will be short-lived. Patients who have sustained relatively minor chest injuries but have undergone abdominal surgery may be in this category. For intubation the nasotracheal route is preferred, because:
1 The tube is more easily secured in position.
2 It is less likely to kink and cannot be chewed by the patient.
3 It causes less salivation and oral sepsis.
4 It is more comfortable and therefore more readily tolerated by the patient.

However, whether the patient has an endotracheal or tracheostomy tube in place, the problems it may create must be recognized and prevented. There is little doubt that intubation increases the risk of upper airway trauma and local infection. This is usually unimportant but rarely it may lead to serious complications, which include nasal or tracheal haemorrhage, tracheal stenosis or dilatation, and tracheo-oesophageal fistula. Most of these are avoidable by attention to detail at the time of intubation or surgery. Good anaesthesia, gentle intubation and skilful surgery are all essential. The longer-term care includes the avoidance of traction on the tubing, the prevention of prolonged hypotension, efficient humidification and, in particular, the use of minimal cuff inflation pressure.

Endotracheal cuff care

In the author's unit tracheal tube cuffs are inflated gradually, and, as the pressure rises, by half millilitre increments, until an airtight seal is obtained. At this point, 0.5 ml air is released and if no leak occurs during positive pressure ventilation a further 0.5 ml is released. When air begins to leak around the tube 0.5 ml is re-injected into the cuff and the pilot tube is occluded. The cuff is not deflated until the tube is removed and the tube is not changed until the patient has recovered—unless the cuff leaks or other technical mishaps occur. Periodic deflation confers no benefits provided that the initial cuff pressure is not excessive, and it may allow secretions which have accumulated above the cuff to pass into the lungs.

Problems after intubation

Intubation reduces the efficiency of coughing and necessitates regular tracheobronchial suction which must be performed gently and aseptically. It probably also increases the risk of systemic sepsis. Any procedure which breaks mucosal or mucocutaneous continuity, particularly in the immunologically compromised patient, is a likely source of systemic sepsis. In addition to tracheal intubation, this includes urethral and intravascular catheterization, but antibiotics should never be used prophylactically since they virtually guarantee the emergence of gram-negative superinfection.

The major problems associated with tracheal intubation and controlled ventilation are technical, namely, ventilator failure, disconnection and obstruction. The inexperienced doctor and nurse naturally assume that tracheal intubation automatically guarantees a patent airway but, sadly, nothing could be further from the truth. Endotracheal tubes and tracheostomy tubes readily become obstructed, kinked, displaced or disconnected from the ventilator or oxygen line.

Endobronchial intubation

A further complication is right endobronchial intubation. This is so common that in the author's unit every patient who is intubated before admission has a chest radiograph taken immediately to establish that the tube is not too long. Although endobronchial intubation can usually be recognized either by observation of the chest movements or with the stethoscope, this does not guarantee safety. Even if the endotracheal or tracheostomy tube is only marginally too long and air can be heard entering the left lung it may make the passage of a suction catheter into the left bronchus impossible, inevitably leading to accumulation of secretions and to atelectasis.

If a patient needs to be intubated while in the unit a simple procedure is adopted which guarantees that endobronchial intubation cannot occur, unless the patient has some congenital tracheobronchial anomaly. Before inserting the tube, a black ring is painted around it with a 'magic marker' just proximal to the cuff (Figure 13). After intubation the black ring must be visible at or just fractionally below the vocal cords. This ensures that only that portion of the tube bearing the cuff is below the cords. If this practice were uniformly adopted, endobronchial intubation would be an exceptional event.

The tip of a tracheostomy tube may enter the right main bronchus if the stoma is made below the third tracheal ring. This condition is very difficult to resolve and it must be avoided at all costs.

If the patient has sustained extensive pulmonary contusions, and in particular if there has been a delay before instituting treatment, with the probability of pneumonia having developed, nasotracheal intubation is less satisfactory than tracheostomy since tracheobronchial suction is much less

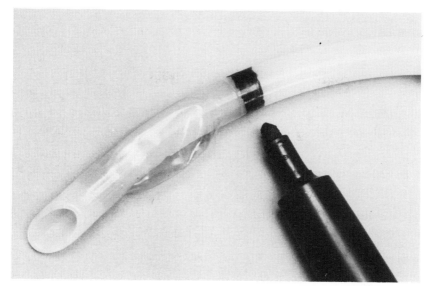

Figure 13. How to avoid endobronchial intubation.

efficient when it is performed via a nasotracheal tube. Straight suction catheters can only rarely and by chance enter the left main bronchus, and coudé tipped catheters cannot easily be directed down nasotracheal tubes. When a coudé catheter is inserted through a tracheostomy tube it can usually be directed into each main bronchus as desired, although the nurse should be instructed to aim the tip into the left side twice out of every three attempts.

Post-intubation care

After intubation the nurse must measure and record the patient's respiratory rate, ventilator cycling pressure and tidal volume at least once each hour since this enables her to recognize underventilation, which is particularly important if the patient is obtunded or receiving systemic narcotics. This will also provide evidence of leaks in the circuit and it will demonstrate any alteration in the patient's compliance.

Tube displacement

Tracheal tube displacement is a potential disaster which must be recognized and corrected immediately. If the patient is receiving controlled ventilation, it is usually followed by the sounds of leakage and may be accompanied by mucus bubbles around the nose, mouth or stoma. The patient will eventually become cyanosed but the nurse must be taught how unreliable, unpredictable and delayed this sign may be. Chest movements disappear although, if he can, the patient will attempt to breathe. The ventilator cycling pressure will change, and if a tidal volume alarm is attached to the expiratory side of the ventilator this will be activated.

If the patient is breathing spontaneously the signs of tube displacement are not so obvious, but if he is conscious he will be able to vocalize or make gurgling noises.

If a tracheostomy tube becomes dislodged into the anterior mediastinum or pre-tracheal tissues whilst the patient is receiving controlled ventilation, chest movements will cease and surgical emphysema will eventually appear.

When any of these signs are noted, the immediate management is laryngoscopy followed by orotracheal intubation and manual ventilation with oxygen. If the patient has a tracheostomy the orotracheal tube must be advanced beyond the stoma and if necessary, pressure applied over it to prevent leakage. If the tracheostomy tube has not been displaced it will be visible on laryngoscopy and some other cause for the alarm must be sought.

If the tracheostomy is less than two days old re-insertion of the tube through the stoma may be difficult because the track is ill-defined, and no attempt should be made to do this until the patient is in a stable condition. A good overhead light, the appropriate retractors and a suction unit must be available. Whenever a patient has a tracheal tube in place, its size should be prominently recorded in the notes and a replacement tube of the same size and another one size smaller must be kept at the patient's bedside for just this type of emergency. Tracheal dilators should always be available for the patient with a tracheostomy.

Partial displacement of tracheal tubes

Occasionally tracheostomy tubes may become partially displaced. Although the external position of the tube may be suggestive this accident is sometimes difficult to recognize. It is usually demonstrated by leakage around the tube and reduction of the measured tidal volume, together with surgical emphysema and difficulty with tracheobronchial toilet. Hopefully this accident will be recognized before the patient's life is put at risk.

Orotracheal and nasotracheal tubes may become partially displaced so that the cuff sits across the vocal cords. This makes the maintenance of an airtight seal difficult, and the attendant usually finds he needs to add progressively more air to the cuff. On laryngoscopy, the upper part of the cuff can be seen bulging above the vocal cords. The initial treatment for these two mishaps is the same as was described for total displacement.

If the medical attendant has any doubt at all as to the correct position of a tracheal tube he must assume that it has been displaced and act accordingly. He must never leave a patient in the care of a nurse or junior member of the medical staff if he feels even faintly unhappy about the patient's airway. If necessary, the patient should be anaesthetized and his entire upper airway examined and the tube replaced. The anaesthetist is, above all other things, the master of the patient's airway and catastrophes which arise due to tube obstruction or misplacement are avoidable.

All nurses who look after very sick or dependent patients must be encouraged to call for help whenever they are concerned and not be afraid to generate a false alarm. It is infinitely better for help to be requested unnecessarily than for it to be called too late.

THE VENTILATORY TREATMENT OF GRADE 3 INJURIES

The reasons for applying positive pressure ventilation are:
1 To permit the effective use of systemic analgesics
2 To achieve satisfactory gas exchange
3 To apply internal pneumatic fixation
4 As an aid to the treatment of non-thoracic injuries

The combined effect of chest-wall and pulmonary parenchymal injuries is to cause hypoventilation (hypercapnia) and ventilation/perfusion ($\dot{V}/\dot{Q}$) imbalance (shunt effect) with consequent hypoxia. More extensive lung injuries which involve a whole lobe or lung produce a true shunt. Controlled ventilation in one form or another is the most effective and least traumatic treatment for injuries of this type, although its efficiency is limited by their extent. If blood and oxygen cannot be brought into apposition, the effects of controlled ventilation are limited. The difference between the haemoglobin dissociation curves for oxygen and carbon dioxide and the latter's greater solubility also influence the results of this form of treatment. It is usually not difficult to correct hypercapnia but hypoxia may be an intractable problem.

Arterial oxygen desaturation due to $\dot{V}/\dot{Q}$ disturbance can usually be corrected by increasing the inspired oxygen concentration (Pio_2), although the Aa oxygen tension gradient may be wide. However, if a true shunt exists, that is, if a significant proportion of the circulating blood volume perfuses totally unventilated lung tissue, the arterial blood will inevitably be desaturated. This cannot be corrected by increasing the Pio_2 in the perfused and ventilated alveoli. Both $\dot{V}/\dot{Q}$ imbalance and true shunt are found in contused and lacerated lung tissue.

The alveolar–arterial oxygen gradient

The difference between the partial pressure of oxygen in the alveolar gas (PAo_2) and that in arterial blood (Pao_2) provides a valuable, though indirect, indication of the true shunt; this is known as the Aa gradient and it should be measured and recorded at frequent intervals during the course of treatment since it gives a good guide to the progress of the lung lesion whether it is caused by trauma, infection or other factors. The alveolar oxygen tension is calculated as follows:

$$PAo_2 = Pio_2 - \frac{Paco_2}{R}$$

where PAo_2 is the partial pressure of oxygen in alvolear gas; Pio_2 is the partial pressure of oxygen in the inspired gas; $Paco_2$ is the partial pressure of carbon dioxide in arterial blood; R is the respiratory exchange ratio, which is usually assumed to be 0.8.

If the patient is very catabolic R may be 0.9. If the patient has been maintained on controlled ventilation for some time and the ventilatory parameters are unchanged, it is acceptable to substitute the Pio_2 for the PAo_2 in this calculation.

The $\dot{V}_E$ *PaCO$_2$* relationship

Figure 14 shows the inverse relationship which exists between the arterial carbon dioxide tension (*Pa*CO$_2$) and minute volume ($\dot{V}_E$); when the $\dot{V}_E$ is doubled, the *Pa*CO$_2$ is halved, and vice versa. It also demonstrates the way in which increasing the physiological dead space reduces the efficiency of ventilation.

The compliance of damaged chest wall and the underlying lung is reduced; the uneven distribution of lung damage causes uneven distribution of ventilation. This is demonstrated in Figure 15, in which the right lung is atelectatic following a unilateral injury, whereas the left lung is undamaged. When positive pressure ventilation is applied most of the fresh gas enters the undamaged (left) lung. The dead space of the left lung is slightly increased by overdistension but the overall effect is moderate hyperventilation so that the carbon dioxide tension of the blood which leaves the left lung is lowered. However, only a fraction of the blood which enters the right lung comes into contact with fresh gas (i.e., there is an extensive shunt) and the distorted chest wall is not supported. Painful spasm of the chest wall muscles reduces its compliance still further.

This represents an extreme but not exceptional case and it is chosen to emphasize that, although it is possible to manipulate the inspired oxygen concentration and tidal and minute volumes, the distribution of the applied gas and the arterial oxygen tension are largely controlled by the extent and

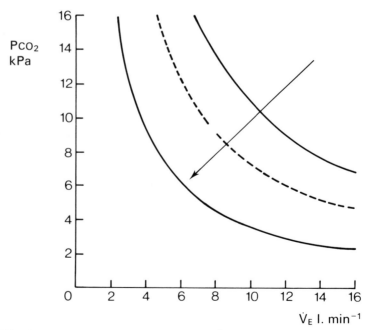

Figure 14. The relationship between minute volume ($\dot{V}_E$) and arterial carbon dioxide tension (PCO$_2$). The arrow shows the effect of reducing the dead space volume. (With thanks to Dr E.A. Cooper.)

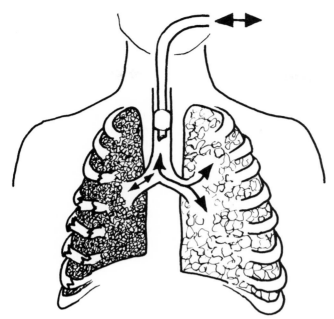

Figure 15. Uneven distribution of compliance due to trauma (or disease) leads to uneven distribution of ventilation. (With thanks to Dr R.A.L. Brewis.)

distribution of pulmonary damage. Only rarely is hypercapnia a serious problem in the ventilated patient, but hypoxia is an ever-present problem. Resistant hypercapnia is an ominous sign, always associated with refractory hypoxia and a poor prognosis.

Choice of ventilatory pattern for IPPV

Many experienced anaesthetists are prepared to make categorical statements as to the best ventilatory wave-form to be used for patients who have suffered extensive thoracic injury. However, from the above introduction it should be obvious that no single system can be the optimum for all types of injury, and only by trial and error, monitored clinically by frequent blood gas analysis and with daily radiography, can the best ventilatory pattern be established for an individual patient.

Frequency dependent compliance

It has been known for many years that a rapid inspiratory gas flow favours the poorly compliant lung whereas a slow gas flow will best ventilate a compliant lung. This is called frequency dependent compliance, and it demonstrates the difficulty of using any set gas flow rate or wave form to ventilate lungs with greatly varied compliance. The state of the conducting airways is also influential: patients with acute or chronic airways obstruction are most satisfactorily ventilated with a slow inspired gas flow rate. It is the author's opinion that for an adult patient with injuries which involve both sides of the chest, the first choice should be:

1 A large tidal volume (800–1000 ml)
2 An accelerating inspiratory flow rate
3 A low respiratory frequency (10–12 bpm)

To facilitate IPPV, initially the patient may need to be heavily sedated and perhaps be given a neuromuscular blocking agent. This is discussed later.

The lowest possible inspired oxygen concentration should be used which will achieve an acceptable PaO_2. The latter depends upon the patient's metabolic rate which in turn is related to the extent of the injury and body temperature, but for the average patient a PaO_2 of 8.0 kPa is quite adequate.

Alternative ventilatory patterns

If when applied with an unsophisticated ventilator this regimen does not have the desired clinical and biochemical effects, the ventilatory wave form can be manipulated. A pattern of rapidly accelerating inspiratory flow followed by an inspiratory hold and rapid deflation, the so-called 'square wave' ventilatory pattern, is favoured by many. Positive end-expiratory pressure (PEEP) is popular in some centres although this, like the square-wave pattern, may accentuate maldistribution since it will force gas into the more compliant parts of the lung while underventilating the damaged areas. The use of PEEP is logical only if the damage is distributed evenly throughout both lungs. PEEP may also increase the risk of barotrauma, by shearing compliant lung against less compliant lung. Its cardiocirculatory effects need no emphasis, although there is evidence which suggests that extensively damaged lung tissue protects the central circulation from the effects of raised intrathoracic pressure.

Alternative methods of treatment

Double lumen tubes

The logical treatment for patients who have severe injuries restricted to one side of the chest includes the passage of a double lumen endobronchial tube and the use of two ventilators (Figure 16). A double lumen tracheostomy tube is also available (Rusche). The PiO_2 and flow patterns can then be adjusted to suit the requirements of each lung. This type of treatment is being assessed in many centres and the preliminary results are encouraging. The theoretical problems of synchronizing the two ventilators appears to be relatively unimportant in practice. A more practical problem is the difficulty of performing effective tracheobronchial toilet through this type of tube.

Intermittent mandatory ventilation

Intermittent mandatory ventilation (IMV) is very popular, but if the patient with extensive chest wall injuries is allowed to breathe against the ventilator, the unstable chest wall will tend to collapse with predictable results which include persistent atelectasis and chest wall deformity. IMV may have a place

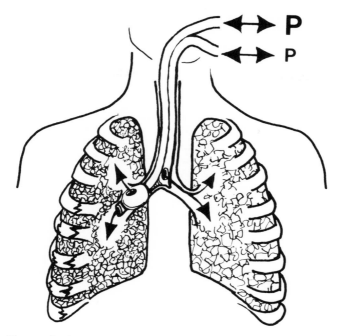

Figure 16. The use of a double-lumen tube and two ventilators to manage unevenly distributed compliance. (With thanks to Dr R.A.L. Brewis.)

when the patient begins to recover from the worst of his injuries, but in the early stages its use defeats the object of the exercise.

High frequency positive pressure ventilation

High frequency positive pressure ventilation (HFPPV) has not been widely used in this situation and no objective opinion of its value can yet be given.

Other aids to effective ventilation

If a single ventilator is used and if, in spite of varying the flow patterns, gross maldistribution is a problem, the attendant can attempt to control this in one of two ways:

1   By applying non-elastic strapping to the *normal* side and thereby reducing its compliance.

2   By nursing the patient with the damaged side uppermost for at least 16 hours out of each 24 hours.

External pressure on the *normal* side will cause ventilation to favour the damaged lung. Usually, patients are nursed on each side alternately, but if the damaged side is favoured, this may help to distribute the inspired gas equally.

   Whichever system of treatment is used, its effects must be monitored and recorded.

Internal pneumatic fixation

This term implies that controlled ventilation encourages the lungs to inflate, corrects the bony deformity and stabilizes the damaged chest wall. Although in most cases the results are very satisfactory, for the reasons given above these objectives are not always fully achieved. Alternative methods, which depend upon surgical fixation, are discussed later in this chapter. If it is decided that controlled ventilation is required, the patient must be discouraged from breathing against the ventilator since this aggravates the chest wall deformity and reduces the efficiency of ventilation. There is also clinical evidence that patients who breathe out of phase with ventilators may develop interstitial pulmonary oedema.

Pneumothorax and haemothorax

When the lungs are inflated against fractured bones there is an obvious risk of pneumothorax and haemothorax which is most likely to occur during the first three to four days after instituting controlled ventilation, although it can occur at any time. Physiotherapy may also increase this hazard, and the physiotherapist must be advised to practise her skills with great gentleness. If a patient's colour deteriorates while he is undergoing controlled ventilation, an erect chest radiograph must be taken as soon as possible (within 15 minutes). However, the clinical signs may indicate that a drainage tube must be inserted without delay and the medical attendant must be prepared to do this without waiting for radiographic confirmation of the diagnosis (page 82).

The indications for discontinuing controlled ventilation

These are:
1 Radiographic resolution of the signs of pulmonary contusion
2 Narrowing of the Aa oxygen tension gradient
3 Diminution or safe control of pain

Of these signs, freedom from pain is particularly important. In other cases, once the underlying pulmonary pathology has cleared, the bony injuries can be expected to resolve. If these are very extensive and include unstable injuries to the sternum, controlled ventilation may need to be continued for two to three weeks. This period is influenced by the extent and significance of other factors, including the patient's pre-incident physical status and the presence of extrathoracic injury. In some centres, intermittent mandatory ventilation (IMV) is used as an aid to the weaning process. Provided that the circuit responds rapidly to the ventilatory demands this can do little harm. On the other hand there is no reliable evidence that IMV facilitates weaning and there is no need to purchase a ventilator which has this option.

In the author's unit the patient is ventilated for the first one to three days with the aid of the combination of pancuronium and an effective analgesic (page 77). Thereafter, the pancuronium is discontinued and gradually over the subsequent days (rarely, weeks) the dose of analgesic is also reduced. When the clinical, laboratory and radiographic evidence suggests that improvement has begun, the patient is allowed to breathe spontaneously for increasing periods while his clinical state, tidal volume and blood gases are monitored. If he becomes tired, or if blood gas analysis indicates that he is not coping, ventilation is re-established until several hours later, or the following day.

The use of antibiotics

Some patients who have sustained extensive chest injuries develop broncho-pneumonia during the course of treatment; many of the others can be expected to produce sputum from which pathogens or commensals can be grown. However, it must be reiterated that antibiotics must be given only if the evidence of bacterial infection (rather than colonization) is convincing. Ill-considered use of antibiotics is a major problem in modern hospital practice. The dangers of all forms of invasive treatment are emphasized throughout this book. All possible efforts must be made to prevent secondary infection, but this can be minimized only if the nurses and medical attendants are fully aware of its dangers.

Pharmacological aids to controlled ventilation

When controlled ventilation is instituted the patient will require sedation and analgesia to reduce anxiety and to provide relief from pain. Very few patients enjoy the sensation of having their respiratory function taken over, and until they become accustomed to it they usually require an anxiolytic drug. The need for analgesia is obvious, but natural or synthetic narcotics are also used because they depress the respiratory centre and simplify the application of IPPV.

Choice of analgesia and sedation

A wide range of drugs is available for this purpose and epidural analgesia can be used from the outset, although if the patient has an endotracheal tube or tracheostomy tube in place he will also need systemic sedation. In the author's department adult patients with grade 3 injuries are given phenoperidine 4 mg hourly by continuous infusion which is reinforced with diazepam emulsion 5–10 mg intravenously six hourly. This regimen is usually required for three to five days, at the end of which the patients can be given progressively less phenoperidine as they become pain-free and accustomed to the ventilator.

Phenoperidine is used because it produces adequate analgesia and respiratory depression with little effect upon the cardiovascular system. It is not a good sedative, and sedation is provided by the addition of diazepam. No signs of pharmacological or psychic dependence have been seen even when this regimen has been used for several weeks, and it does not appear to cause suprarenal suppression. The most troublesome side-effects are delayed gastric emptying and constipation, which sometimes create the need for parenteral nutrition. Some patients develop intestinal hurry when the phenoperidine infusion is discontinued.

Alternatives to phenoperidine

If phenoperidine is not available any similar narcotic agent may be used. If the patient is unlikely to need analgesics for more than a few days, an infusion of morphine or papaveretum can be used as an alternative to phenoperidine until he becomes accustomed to the ventilator. However, the amounts required sometimes have undesirable cardiocirculatory side-effects and the potential problem of addiction must be considered, although this is remote. It is usual to start with a 10–20 mg intravenous bolus injection followed by 10–15 mg hourly by continuous infusion. After 12 hours the infusion rate may be reduced. This drug also causes constipation and may delay gastric emptying.

The use of muscle relaxants

Muscle relaxants must never be used in the absence of adequate sedation, but not infrequently a patient who is pain-free, and with acceptable blood gases and hydrogen ion status makes inappropriate respiratory efforts. These can usually be overcome by temporarily increasing the alveolar ventilation and thereby causing hypocapnia. When spontaneous ventilatory efforts cease, the alveolar ventilation can be reduced gradually without causing the patient to breathe against the ventilator. An alternative method is to insert an extra dead space into the ventilator circuit and then increase the patient's tidal volume by the volume of the dead space—usually 200–250 ml. The resulting increase in chest distension frequently inhibits voluntary movements, with no effect upon the arterial carbon dioxide tension.

If neither of these methods is successful and the patient is still breathing against the machine and aggravating his chest wall instability a muscle relaxant should be used for 24–48 hours. Pancuronium 4 mg/h by infusion is usually given, but only after the patient has been told what is about to happen so that if, by mischance, the analgesia or sedation wears off he will understand why he cannot move. Obviously this is a most undesirable circumstance, and relaxants should be avoided or used for as short a time as possible. There should be no need to state that when heavy sedation, with or without relaxants, is prescribed the medical attendant must be able to place absolute reliance on the nursing staff and the ventilator circuitry.

THE PROBLEM OF OCCULT INJURIES

Intra-abdominal injuries

Some of the more obvious injuries which are associated with chest trauma are discussed later in the chapter, but patients who have suffered major chest trauma may also have suffered intra-abdominal injuries which are not apparent when the decision to sedate, paralyse and ventilate the patient has to be taken. The diagnosis of delayed visceral rupture or of splenic or hepatic injury may be very difficult when the patient is sedated and/or paralysed. If there is any question of such an injury being present, a sympathetic surgeon must be found who is willing to try to exclude it before long-term ventilation is begun. Peritoneal lavage is discussed on page 72; although it is a valuable technique it may not necessarily establish the presence of ischaemic but intact bowel. One of the author's surgical colleagues is quite prepared to perform a laparotomy in these circumstances and he is not too concerned if the results are negative. If, during the course of his treatment, a patient has a persisting paralytic ileus with abdominal distension, it is very comforting to remember that he has had a laparotomy which has either excluded intra-abdominal injury or treated it appropriately.

It was stated earlier that the combination of serious chest injuries with abdominal sepsis carries a high mortality; this can only be increased if the diagnosis is delayed. In many units, a laparotomy is always performed before long-term IPPV is commenced on patients with possible internal injuries.

Aortic arch rupture

The aortic arch ruptures where its mobile and fixed segments meet, on one or other side of the vertebral column. This is one of the most lethal complications of chest wall trauma but at the same time, provided the patient reaches hospital alive, it is relatively easy to treat. If the patient is more than 50 years of age the injury is usually immediately fatal because of the rigidity of the aorta, but younger patients may survive with partial rupture for hours, days or longer.

Clinical features

Aortic arch rupture is usually due to violent forward flexion of the upper thorax which is often associated with fractures of posterior segments of the second or third rib and wedge fractures of upper thoracic vertebrae. These signs are so suggestive that in their presence an arch aortogram should be performed, with a cardiothoracic team poised to perform an immediate thoracotomy. Aortography is potentially lethal in this condition and, if it is available, digital vascular imaging (DVI) provides a less dangerous technique for identifying aortic arch rupture.

The diagnosis is also suggested if there is a difference of more than 20 mm Hg when the blood pressure is measured in both arms. This examination should be routinely performed on every patient with chest trauma (or multiple injuries). If the rupture is on the left side of the arch beyond the left subclavian artery, the femoral pulses may be diminished or absent.

Classically, the chest radiograph shows widening of the superior mediastinum and pleural fluid may be noted, but these signs are not always present and the diagnosis can then be confirmed only if an arch aortogram is performed.

Treatment

Treatment may involve cardiopulmonary bypass, although a left ventricle-to-descending aorta cannula has been designed to eliminate the need for full bypass. If the diagnosis is made in time the results are quite good, but if not the patient usually dies within a few hours, although more prolonged survival is not unknown; occasionally a false aneurysm forms which is recognized only long after the event.

Pericardial tamponade

This condition is due to the accumulation of fluid (usually blood) in the pericardial sac, preventing ventricular filling and leading to a rapidly progressive fall in cardiac output. It may be caused by a penetrating injury, but it most frequently follows moving vehicle accidents when it is caused by the victim's forward progress being abruptly halted by the steering column. Often the result is sudden death from cardiac damage but patients may survive for many hours. The bleeding originates from either pericardial or epicardial vessels: rarely from small cardiac tears. Although the presenting evidence is clinical, the diagnosis may be suggested by radiographic evidence of cardiac enlargement in the absence of cardiocirculatory symptoms. If there is time, it can be confirmed by ultrasonic scan.

Clinical signs

The clinical signs of pericardial tamponade are:
1 Dyspnoea or tachypnoea
2 Fall in cardiac output
3 Engorgement of head, neck and upper limb veins
4 Pulsus paradoxus

If the patient is conscious he usually complains of breathlessness and of an oppressive central chest discomfort and a feeling of impending death.

Recognition and treatment

The treatment is both very easy and very gratifying since the improvement is so dramatic, provided the diagnosis is correct. A 14 gauge (or larger) cannula such as a Medicut or Abbocath fitted to a 20 ml syringe is inserted through the left fifth intercostal space 1 cm from the sternal edge and advanced slowly, aspirating all the way. With an average-sized adult, at a depth of 1.5–2.0 cm, blood can be aspirated freely, and when the syringe and inner cannula are removed, blood is ejected in a pulsatile manner. This can be disconcerting, and if the cannula moves very vigorously with pulsation it is remotely possible that the right ventricle has been transfixed, but this is usually accompanied by runs of ectopic beats.

A few millilitres of blood should be placed in a glass tube and watched for four minutes to see if it clots: pericardial blood is usually defibrinated and does not clot. If the physical signs are convincing and the patient appears to be in danger of death, there is no need to wait for the results of this test. A three-way tap is fitted to the end of the cannula and aspiration commenced. Most patients with tamponade improve rapidly after 100–300 ml blood are removed but aspiration should continue until the sac is dry. Alternatively, a soft intravascular catheter can be introduced into the pericardial sac via the cannula and allowed to drain spontaneously. If the bleeding persists and only temporary relief is obtained a cardiac surgeon should be consulted since it may be necessary to perform a pericardiectomy or open drainage procedure.

If the diagnosis is incorrect and this volume of blood is accidentally removed from the right ventricle no harm results.

Myocardial contusion

Patient who have suffered blunt thoracic trauma may sustain a variety of other cardiac injuries. In many cases death occurs instantly or before help is available, but myocardial contusions, which can give rise to delayed problems, may occur. These may be suggested by the ECG signs which are non-specific but include ST segment and T wave abnormalities suggestive of myocardial ischaemia. Tachydysrhythmias are common.

If any of these signs is noted, an ultrasound scan should be performed since pericardial tamponade is a constant hazard. With the possible exception of creatinine phosphokinase isoenzyme (CPK), the measurement of cardiac enzymes is of little diagnostic value in the traumatized patient, and proof of the existence of myocardial contusions can be obtained only at thoracotomy or at autopsy. Nevertheless, if the evidence is suggestive, the patient should be given either lignocaine or disopyramide (Rhythmodan) by infusion since ventricular tachycardia and ventricular fibrillation commonly occur after myocardial contusion.

Pneumothorax, haemothorax

Probably as many as 20% of all patients with chest injuries show evidence of a pneumothorax on admission to hospital, and a significant number develop this complication after admission—either spontaneously or as a result of treatment. It is often accompanied by haemothorax. Everyone who is concerned with the care of injured patients must be able to recognize and treat these conditions.

Clinical signs

The clinical signs of pneumothorax may be obvious, although patients with low pressure pneumothorax frequently have few diagnostic signs. These are often obscured or difficult to elicit because of the pain, dyspnoea and ventilatory limitations caused by the chest wall injury together with underlying pulmonary parenchymal damage. If the patient is receiving IPPV the diagnosis may be even more difficult.

If the patient is breathing spontaneously, examination *may* reveal:
1 Cyanosis
2 Dyspnoea and tachypnoea
3 Tracheal deviation *towards* the injured side
4 Reduced chest movement
5 Increased resonance to percussion
6 Diminished vocal resonance
7 Diminished air entry

Occasionally the patient may cough up blood-stained sputum.

Tension pneumothorax

If the pneumothorax is under tension, the respiratory and cardiocirculatory signs are more marked. Acute dyspnoea, cyanosis and greatly reduced cardiac output are accompanied by tracheal deviation *away* from the injured side together with the other signs listed above. In either case, if the patient is able, he may complain of a sharp chest pain on the appropriate side.

If the patient is receiving controlled ventilation the position of the trachea may be influenced by the tracheal tube and breath sounds may be transmitted across the midline from the other side, making the diagnosis more difficult.

A high index of suspicion is necessary at all times and, in an emergency, it may be necessary to act on the physical signs alone or together with clinical and laboratory evidence of hypoxia. Wherever possible a chest radiograph should first be taken since patients with extensive chest injuries frequently present very misleading physical signs; the erect position is preferable since pleural fluid is not always clearly visible in supine films. In addition, the position of the diaphragm may be obscured and occasionally a 'false' pneumothorax may confuse the attendant: this appearance, most commonly seen in the elderly, is produced by a posterior skin fold and it should be easily distinguished from the lung edge by the presence of pulmonary vascular markings beyond it.

Not infrequently, patients develop bilateral pneumothorax after chest injuries and their recognition is extremely difficult without a chest radiograph, since the signs are the same on both sides. The only way to prevent this incident from resulting in disaster is to keep its possibility in mind.

Treatment

If the diagnosis of pneumothorax is confirmed its significance must be considered before a chest drainage tube is inserted. If the patient is breathing spontaneously and is not hypoxic, and the pneumothorax occupies less than one-fifth (estimated) of the thoracic cavity, it may be felt that the risks of inserting a chest tube outweigh its advantages, particularly if the patient is pain-free, breathing and coughing freely and has an acceptable Pao_2. However, if these criteria are not met, or if the signs do not resolve inside 24 hours, or if the patient requires surgical treatment under general anaesthesia, a tube should be inserted. The pneumothorax may enlarge or develop high tension whilst the patient is anaesthetized. These possibilities should always be borne in mind if an injured patient requires general anaesthesia.

If the patient with a pneumothorax is receiving controlled ventilation a chest tube should always be inserted since it will probably increase in size and embarrass the circulation. The radiographic signs of tension pneumothorax include displacement of the mediastinum *away* from the affected collapsed lung and downward displacement of the diaphragm on the same side. Very occasionally, if the patient is receiving controlled ventilation the diaphragm may actually be inverted.

Chest drainage

The optimum site for insertion of chest drains is disputed, but the author believes this should be the mid-axillary or posterior axillary line in the sixth or seventh intercostal space. The traditional anterior 'medical' site is useless for the drainage of fluid, and if the tube is inserted behind the posterior axillary line it readily becomes kinked. The patient's position in bed and his ability to move about are also restricted.

The type of tube used is a matter of personal preference, but it should be of an adequate size; whichever site or tube is used, unless the patient is unconscious, a very generous amount of local anaesthetic solution must be infiltrated since it is a very painful procedure. The costal periosteum appears to be particularly sensitive and an attempt should always be made to infiltrate the local anaesthetic very close to it.

Complications of chest drainage

The problems associated with chest drainage include:
1 Unnecessary insertion
2 Haemorrhage
3 Sepsis
4 Fistula formation
5 Subphrenic insertion

The first of these may occasionally be unavoidable if the clinician feels impelled to insert a drain without first obtaining a chest radiograph. It may cause a pneumothorax, sometimes accompanied by bleeding. Haemorrhage from the insertion of a chest drain in the site recommended is very rarely severe, whereas the anterior approach may be associated with heavy bleeding from the internal mammary artery. Exceptionally, an intercostal vessel is damaged but this rarely causes significant bleeding. Sepsis can be avoided only by paying strict attention to aseptic insertion and maintenance, and the tube should be removed as soon as it has fulfilled its function.

Bronchopleural fistula. If the patient is receiving controlled ventilation the tear in the lung may be slow to heal, and much of the tidal volume may be lost and gas exchange may be inadequate. If it does not show rapid signs of resolution, a thoracotomy and repair are necessary; this may occasionally demonstrate that the initial pneumothorax was caused by bronchial injury and bronchopleural fistula.

Subphrenic insertion. It is surprisingly easy to insert a chest drain below the diaphragm, particularly if the procedure is performed with the patient supine and without the aid of a chest radiograph. If the latter is taken with the patient erect, the diaphragm can usually be identified but if there is any doubt as to its position, and particularly if the patient's abdomen is distended, the drain should be inserted through a higher intercostal space. It is a good practice first to enter the pleural cavity with the needle through which the local anaesthetic is being injected. If air or blood can be aspirated freely, it is usually safe to insert a drainage tube through the same site. However, if the needle is inserted below the diaphragm and the peritoneal cavity contains blood this test is not reliable.

Removal of chest drains

After the lung has been fully expanded for 24 hours, bubbles have ceased to emerge from the underwater drain, and any drainage of blood has stopped, a clamp should be placed across the tube. Four hours later an erect chest radiograph should be taken to determine whether or not the pneumothorax has recurred. If not the tube may be removed.

Injuries to the clavicle

These are usually regarded as being of little functional importance, but the clavicle may be fractured together with anterior rib fractures on the same side and increase the degree of chest wall instability. The clavicle may also be fractured following direct injury to the supraclavicular region which may involve the brachial plexus. Rarely the roots of the phrenic nerve are damaged, which may lead to diaphragmatic paralysis. This may cause respiratory difficulty which is explained only by the finding of elevation of the diaphragm on plain x-ray, and confirmed by screening. If the diaphragm is the only part of the chest involved, it should not cause severe incapacity unless the patient has a pre-existing respiratory problem.

Surgical treatment of chest injuries

Chest wall injuries are still treated surgically in some centres. The treatment ranges from the application of traction to the unstable chest wall to the open reduction of multiple rib fractures, with fixation by wires, plates or a wide variety of clamps. In the author's experience the place for such manoeuvres is strictly limited.

If the patient requires surgical treatment for open chest wall injuries or because of intrathoracic damage, it is logical to attempt to stabilize the chest wall afterwards. The method which is used for this purpose depends upon the surgeon's personal choice but in most cases the result is not good. Surgical wounds become infected, wires bend, plates loosen and clamps slip. The surgical approach to chest wall injuries involves the patient in very extensive skin mobilization and prolonged traumatic surgery, with the risks of haemorrhage and infection, to say nothing of a very painful post-operative course. If the patient has extensive pulmonary contusions or lacerations he will still require controlled ventilation with added oxygen for a variable period, and the main objective of surgery, which is to avoid such ministrations, is lost.

Prevention of permanent deformity

The other objective, which is to correct the bony deformity which may occasionally give rise to permanent disfigurement, should be seriously considered. If the patient is young and has very extensive chest wall fractures with deformities which do not respond quickly to controlled ventilation, surgical treatment may be considered. However, in the author's experience, only the elderly are left with much chest wall deformity and the surgical treatment of chest wall injuries in patients over the age of 70 years is a hazardous procedure.

Extracorporeal membrane oxygenation

Extracorporeal membrane oxygenation (ECMO) has been used to treat all types of acute and subacute respiratory failure, including pulmonary trauma. The results have been uniformly bad, since the natural history of the disturbance implies that any form of extracorporeal assistance will be needed for at least seven days. The maintenance of ECMO for more than a few days is a technical and administrative nightmare and the cost is exorbitant. In the author's limited experience with ECMO it has been possible to prolong survival for up to five days, but the patient has always died either from haemorrhage in the lungs or elsewhere, or from failure of oxygenation.

References

Carlon, G.C., Cole Ray, R.R.T., Klain, M. & McCormack, P.M. (1980) High frequency positive pressure ventilation in management of a patient with bronchopleural fistula. *Anesthesiology*, **52**, 160–162.

Dajee, A., Schepps, D. & Hurley, E.J. (1981) Diaphragmatic injuries. *Surgery, Gynecology and Obstetrics*, **153**, 31–32.

Kirsh, M.M. & Sloan, H. (1977) *Blunt Chest Trauma*. 247 pp. Boston: Little, Brown and Company.

Lloyd, J.W., Crampton Smith, A. & O'Connor, B.T. (1965) Classification of chest injuries as an aid to treatment. *British Medical Journal*, **1**, 1518–1520.

Trinkle, J.K., Richardson, J.D. et al (1975) Management of flail chest without mechanical ventilation. *Annals of Thoracic Surgery*, **19**, 355–359.

Williams, W.G. & Smith, R.E. (1977) *Trauma of the Chest*. 266 pp. Bristol: John Wright and Sons.

Wilson, J.M., Thomas, A.N., Goodman, P.C. & Lewis, F.R. (1978) Severe chest trauma: morbidity implication of first and second rib fracture in 120 patients. *Archives of Surgery*, **113**, 846–849.

5

The Adult Respiratory Distress Syndrome

For the purpose of this chapter the adult respiratory distress syndrome (ARDS) is defined as acute or subacute respiratory failure characterized by progressive hypoxia and terminal hypercapnia, associated with non-thoracic trauma, extensive surgical operations and systemic sepsis. It is also known as shock lung, Da-Nang wet lung and post-traumatic respiratory insufficiency.

INCIDENCE

For many years it has been realized that as many as 30% of the patients who die after major trauma do so from progressive respiratory failure. In most cases the cause of death is either bronchopneumonia or aspiration pneumonia, but occasionally these labels do not fit the clinical picture. The problem is made more complex by the fact that the lungs can react in only a limited number of ways to a wide variety of insults. Often the result is that at the autopsy the pathologist is unable to determine what the initiating cause of the patient's respiratory problem was. Occasionally clear-cut evidence of aspiration pneumonia is provided by the identification of polymorph infiltration and foreign body giant cells, and patients who die from primary bacterial pneumonia offer no diagnostic challenge. However, with modern methods of treatment, patients can be kept alive for long periods after having suffered insults to the respiratory system or elsewhere which only a few years ago would have been fatal within hours or days. This has given rise to the term 'pathology of progress' which acknowledges the fact that many of the pathology textbook descriptions of disease are obscured by resuscitation and prolongation of the process of dying.

Autopsy findings

At autopsy the lungs of patients who die after trauma are often found to be heavy, airless and waterlogged. Invariably there are areas of pneumonic consolidation and, in some cases, abscess formation. Histologically there is evidence of infection with polymorph exudation. The alveolar wall is lined with hyaline material which may contain fibrin; it is usually thickened and oedematous and fibroblasts may be identifiable. Fibrosis is a prominent feature of ARDS if the patient survives five to ten days after its initiation. Type

1 pneumocytes are replaced by Type 2 pneumocytes, which are responsible for the formation of surfactant.

Intravascular emboli composed of platelets and leucocytes may be seen, and at a later stage the vessels may be completely occluded by amorphous material. The pathologist's opinion as to the cause of death usually relies upon the evidence of bronchopneumonia but may refer to 'infected pulmonary oedema', 'oxygen toxicity', 'fat embolism' or 'ARDS'.

DIAGNOSTIC CRITERIA

It is the author's opinion that ARDS should be a diagnosis by exclusion. The term should not be used if there is evidence of primary bacterial or viral pneumonia, aspiration of gastric contents, or inhalation of smoke or other chemicals. Similarly, if the initiating cause is direct pulmonary trauma or pulmonary oedema due to either heart failure or to hypoalbuminaemia, or if the disturbance begins in one lung and remains unilateral for more than 24 hours, the diagnostic tag 'ARDS' should not be used.

Pathophysiology

Having excluded the conditions mentioned above, the evidence at present available suggests that the lesion originates in the pulmonary arterioles and capillaries. The sequence of events is thought to be as follows:

1 Physical trauma with extensive tissue damage leads to blood hypercoagulability with an increase in platelet adhesiveness.

2 The platelets aggregate with leucocytes and are filtered out in the terminal pulmonary arterioles where they adhere to the vessel wall, which may already have been damaged by endotoxin.

3 The aggregates obstruct the pulmonary vessels and cause reflex hypertension. As the platelets lyse they release substances which include histamine, serotonin (5-hydroxytryptamine), and thromboxane (an arachidonic acid derivative).

4 The damaged vessel wall releases prostaglandin F_2 alpha.

These substances have both local and systemic effects, causing bronchospasm, vasodilatation and hypotension, and may initiate DIC (page 94). They also increase pulmonary capillary permeability, causing interstitial oedema, and may be in part responsible for the generalized capillary leak syndrome described in Chapter 2.

In addition to its many other effects, endotoxin from gram-negative organisms probably increases capillary hydrostatic pressure, encouraging the leakage of intravascular fluid and protein.

Cardiocirculatory effects

The combined effects of thromboembolism and arteriolar spasm bring about a sustained rise in right ventricular end-diastolic pressure and greatly increase cardiac work. This may ultimately lead to right ventricular failure, which in turn increases the danger of hepatic and renal failure. An otherwise unexplained rise in central venous pressure or pulmonary wedge pressure may be attributable to post-capillary venous spasm.

Haematological effects

Other factors which may contribute are secondary to septicaemia, with or without hypoproteinaemia. Septicaemia is the best known trigger for disseminated intravascular coagulation (DIC, consumptive coagulopathy) (page 94) and it is always accompanied by some degree of impairment of respiratory and renal function. Thromboxane is only one of the many agents which may be responsible.

Platelet coagulation due to trauma may predispose to septicaemia through saturation of the reticuloendothelial system. The activation of complement is believed to be an essential link in the chain of events which leads to ARDS. Complement C_5 alpha, which encourages leucocyte aggregation, is activated by trauma, systemic sepsis and acute pancreatitis. It may also cause the release of toxic free oxygen radicals which, experimentally, have been demonstrated to cause pulmonary capillary damage.

Hypoalbuminaemia

The part played by hypoalbuminaemia has already been alluded to. Albumin is responsible for the greater part of the plasma oncotic pressure, and if the level falls below 30 g/l systemic and pulmonary oedema may develop, although patients with hypoalbuminaemia due to starvation are not always oedematous and this is not the only factor involved. The pulmonary hydrostatic pressure is considerably lower than that in systemic capillaries and the elements of the Starling equation (Figure 4) are tilted in favour of fluid reabsorption. However, if the serum albumin falls markedly the risk of pulmonary oedema increases, particularly when it is combined with pulmonary hypertension.

There is experimental and clinical evidence which suggests that damaged alveolar capillaries are more than usually permeable to albumin which initially leaks into the pulmonary interstitium and ultimately into the alveoli.

Evidence obtained from studies of high altitude pulmonary oedema indicates that activation of the autonomic nervous system increases pulmonary capillary hydrostatic pressure, and bacterial endotoxin may have a similar effect. These observations may have implications for treatment.

Pulmonary microembolism

In Chapter 2 it was suggested that the transfusion of banked blood may have many disadvantages and the use of blood filters was discussed. As stored blood ages, the mass of aggregated white cells, platelets and denatured proteins within the blood pack increases. Those aggregates which are small enough to pass through the standard 70 μm infusion-set filter may be trapped in the pulmonary arterioles and have the same effects as aggregates which are formed in the body. This factor is often quoted as a major cause of ARDS, although the widespread use of blood filters has not appreciably reduced the incidence of the syndrome.

Pulmonary lymphatics

The pulmonary lymphatics play a vital part in the removal of transuded fluids from the interstitium of both the normal and damaged lung and it is widely believed that failure of the lymphatic system is an early feature of ARDS. The lymphatic channels contain valves which maintain undirectional flow. This may have relevance to the use of PEEP in the treatment of ARDS, and will be discussed later (page 93).

Acute pancreatitis and ARDS

Patients with haemorrhagic pancreatitis are invariably found to have a subnormal arterial oxygen tension. Although there are many possible causes for this, in most cases the respiratory abnormality is identical with ARDS due to trauma and sepsis. It has been postulated that the combination of the elevated level of proteolytic enzymes and complement activation are responsible.

CLINICAL PRESENTATION

ARDS takes many forms but typically presents in the following way:

Day 1 The patient, who was previously fit and may be of any age, sustains major injuries to the abdomen, pelvis and lower limbs. On admission to hospital he is shocked and requires a large volume fluid infusion. Initially this consists of crystalloid and plasma protein fraction and (perhaps) some compatible though uncross-matched and unfiltered blood. After resuscitation he is taken to the operating room where he undergoes prolonged abdominal and orthopaedic surgery and further blood transfusions are given. Laparotomy shows that he has some peritoneal soiling due to small bowel rupture. A urinary catheter and an intravenous line are inserted and at the end of three hours of surgery the patient is returned to the ITU receiving IPPV via a nasotracheal tube. The portable chest radiograph taken when the patient returns from the operating room is unremarkable. It is noted that his Aa gradient is rather wider than normal but he is not hypoxic and at no time on Day 1 is any anxiety felt about his respiratory state.

Day 2 The patient appears to be well. The cardiocirculatory parameters are stable. He is allowed to breathe spontaneously and since he maintains satisfactory gas exchange he is extubated. After extubation, he is noted to have a rapid respiratory rate while breathing oxygen-enriched air, and when his blood gases are re-checked he is found to be hyperventilating (Pa_{CO_3}3.5 kPa). There is a small amount of blood-stained fluid in the abdominal drains, his abdomen is distended, he has no bowel sounds but his urine output is satisfactory. Chest radiograph demonstrates elevation of both diaphragms and some basal linear atelectasis.

Day 3   The patient is less well. He has a slightly elevated temperature (37.8°) and a tachycardia. His abdomen is tense and tender. He is still hyperventilating but the Base Excess has fallen and his pH is now within the normal range. The Aa gradient is wider than before. The chest radiograph shows some fluffy shadowing at both lung bases with a suggestion of pulmonary venous engorgement. It is decided he requires further respiratory assistance so he is sedated and re-intubated, and controlled ventilation is re-applied. Although his blood gases and hydrogen ion status are within normal limits and despite heavy sedation the patient continues to breathe against the ventilator, so he is given a muscle relaxant. It is noted that his platelet count has fallen to $60 \times 10^9/l$ and that his prothrombin time is 60% of normal.

Day 4   The patient is very ill indeed. His temperature is 38°C and pulse rate 100 bpm. In spite of fluid restriction and the use of diuretics, the ventilator cycling pressure has risen and chest radiography shows widespread patchy shadowing in both lung fields and some fluid in the horizontal fissure; the Aa P_{O_2} tension gradient is very wide and the patient's flanks are beginning to look oedematous. In spite of increasing the inspired oxygen fraction to 0.7 he is hypoxic and 10 cm PEEP is applied. The Pa_{CO_2} is now at the upper limit of normal although the tidal volume has been increased to 900 ml and the respiratory rate to 14 bpm. The Base Excess is -8 mmol/l. The urine osmolality has fallen and the plasma urea and creatinine have risen. The platelet count is $60 \times 10^9/l$ and the leucocyte count is $12 \times 10^9/l$. The serum albumin is 26 g and he is given two units of low salt albumin. The sputum is scanty and purulent.

Day 5 All of the parameters measured show that the deterioration has continued. The patient is now frankly acidaemic due to a combination of hypercapnia and early renal failure. The Pa_{O_2} has dropped still further and he is clinically jaundiced. The midline surgical wound is bleeding slightly. The prothrombin time has fallen to 50% of normal, the fibrinogen level is 1 g/l and the level of fibrin degradation products is 200 $\mu g/ml$. He is given three units of fresh frozen plasma.

Day 6   The patient has two episodes of asystole due to intractable hypoxia.

Day 7   The patient dies.

The autopsy examinations confirm the presence of the injuries which were previously recognized, but in addition there is a small pelvic abscess from which a variety of organisms is isolated. The pulmonary pathology is as described on page 86.
    This melancholy sequence has variants, but in most reported series, and in the author's own experience, the mortality rate for this condition is at least 50% although the patients do not always die from hypoxia. By the third or fourth day of the illness many patients show obvious signs of septicaemia with acute renal failure.

EFFECTS OF ARDS ON BLOOD GASES AND HYDROGEN ION REGULATION

The diagnostic features of ARDS are said to be hypoxia together with inappropriate hyperventilation, that is, hyperventilation which is not due to pain, anxiety or acidaemia. However, by the nature of the condition, these cannot always be excluded, but at the outset hyperventilation (respiratory alkalaemia) is often accompanied by non-respiratory alkalaemia which can usually be explained by the large volume of stored blood the patient has received.

Although initially blood transfusion causes a mild transient acidaemia, the citrate anticoagulant is metabolized to bicarbonate and by the following day most patients have a non-respiratory alkalaemia. Other factors which may be involved include the use of sodium bicarbonate during resuscitation and continuous nasogastric aspiration.

As the condition progresses the patient develops a non-respiratory acidaemia which may be partially due to renal impairment, although occasionally lactic acidosis is identified. Acidaemia normally causes hyperventilation, and although by this time the patient is usually undergoing controlled ventilation the effect of acidaemia is recognizable from the patient's attempts to breathe out of phase with the machine. A coagulation defect or frank DIC is also commonly present.

INVESTIGATION OF ARDS

The investigations which give the most useful information about the progress of the disease have been mentioned at various stages earlier. These include:
1 Chest radiography
2 Arterial blood gases and hydrogen ion status
3 Accurate measurement of Pio_2 and Aa gradient
4 Mixed venous Po_2
5 Plasma lactate level
6 Comprehensive, detailed and accurate fluid balance records
7 Full coagulation screen
8 Total protein and albumin levels
9 Serum amylase
10 Serum ionized calcium
11 Liver function tests
12 Full microbiological screen.

In some centres, many of the toxic agents mentioned earlier can be measured. These include prostaglandin F_2 alpha, thromboxane and endotoxin levels. More specialized investigations may be used to establish the presence of pulmonary thromboembolism. If a suitable radio-opaque contrast medium (such as 'angioconray') is injected into a pulmonary artery catheter, some of it will still be recognizable on a chest radiograph taken two hours later. Similarly, if ^{131}I fibrinogen is injected, scattered areas of radioactivity can still be identified in the chest many minutes after the injection.

Most of the investigations listed should be repeated daily so that the progress of the illness can be recognized and recorded. Blood gas measurement and the Aa gradient are the most reliable indicators of the progress of the condition and may need to be performed hourly, or even more frequently, during periods of rapid change or in an attempt to assess the effects of treatment. This may demand the insertion of an arterial cannula but it should be removed after 72 hours at most since the hazards of this procedure are increased with time. Invasive monitoring should be avoided if possible since the treatment of the condition does not depend upon it and any type of intravascular monitoring is potentially traumatic and increases the risk of infection.

PREVENTION OF ARDS

In the present state of knowledge it is almost certainly impractical to discuss this topic. The sequence of events which provokes ARDS is probably set in motion immediately after the injury but various methods of prevention have been described. These include full heparinization as soon as the definitive surgery is completed, the use of prostaglandin inhibitors such as ibuprofen, indomethacin or dazoxibens, and the use of massive doses of corticosteroids to inhibit leucocyte aggregation, as soon as the patient is admitted to hospital. Unfortunately, since at present there is no way to predict that a patient will develop ARDS, there is as yet no evidence that any prophylactic measure can prevent its occurrence. Corticosteroids have long since been abandoned by most experienced clinicians. The use of prostaglandin inhibitors appears to be logical while having the smallest number of side-effects, but it will require a very prolonged multicentre controlled trial before their effects can be assessed.

Since fragments from stored blood may play some part in the development of ARDS, microfilters should be used whenever large volume infusions are given.

The prevention of infection has been referred to in many of the preceding sections. There is no doubt that systemic sepsis plays a major part—if not the most important one—in the development of ARDS, and every effort should be made to prevent its occurrence, or at least to treat it quickly and effectively when it occurs.

Prevention or treatment of pulmonary oedema

In Chapter 2 it was stated that fluid overload was a constant hazard after emergency resuscitation, and there is no doubt that many cases of ARDS are, at least in part, due to this. Overload cannot always be avoided in the acute phase of treatment but as soon as the patient is admitted to the ITU a retrospective assessment of fluid balance must be attempted. If he has received overgenerous infusions of crystalloids or other fluids, it is justifiable to give one dose of frusemide 40 mg intravenously. The resulting diuresis sometimes makes an appreciable difference to the ventilator cycling pressure and narrows the Aa gradient, indicating that intrapulmonary water has been mobilized. If the diuresis is short-lived and there is reliable evidence of overload, a second dose of diuretic may be given. The use of frusemide in ARDS is analogous to its use in direct pulmonary trauma: it is intended to help the lungs, not the kidneys.

Thereafter the fluid balance must be very carefully controlled and it is probably safer to err on the side of underhydration than to run the risk of provoking pulmonary oedema.

THE TREATMENT OF ARDS

The aims of treatment are to achieve satisfactory gas exchange with minimal damage to other organs and to identify and treat the underlying cause.

The mortality rate of patients with ARDS is greater than 50%, but death is not always due to respiratory failure as most of the other organs—including the heart, liver and kidneys—are usually damaged to a greater or lesser degree. The prevention or treatment of systemic sepsis is a major problem; this is discussed in greater detail in Chapter 2, but the hypothetical case report which is given at the beginning of this chapter demonstrates how many potential sources of infection are created by treatment in the operating room and ITU.

Controlled ventilation

Hypoxia is the most immediate problem in most cases of ARDS. Hypercapnia is a late and almost invariably a pre-terminal event.

Controlled ventilation with oxygen-enriched air is the standard method of treatment, and in most cases PEEP is used at some stage. Many experienced clinicians use PEEP from the moment the diagnosis is made, whereas others with equal experience use it only if it becomes impossible to maintain an acceptable Pao_2 without an unacceptably high Pio_2 being applied. In the first group there are many who believe that PEEP forces the excess intrapulmonary water back into the systemic circulation, although most recent reviews have established that this does not happen; there is an increasingly large body of data which suggests that PEEP actually increases lung water. The potential importance of the pulmonary lymphatic valves was referred to earlier. Their presence implies that PEEP should augment undirectional lymph flow and help to clear oedema, but experimental work with pulmonary lymphatic fistulae does not support this thesis.

The effects of PEEP on small airway closure, functional residual capacity and ventilation/perfusion ratios are variable, but in most cases it increases the Pao_2 by an unpredictable amount while at the same time increasing ventilation/perfusion inequality and usually causing a small rise in $Paco_2$.

'Best PEEP'

'Best PEEP' describes the technique by which positive end-expiratory pressure is applied in stages, whilst all of its effects, both beneficial and potentially harmful, are monitored and recorded. Ideally the arterial and mixed venous oxygen tensions are measured whilst the cardiac output is continuously recorded so that the amount of oxygen actually delivered to the tissues is determined. The level which is eventually applied is a compromise between the minimal Fio_2 and the optimal Pao_2.

If PEEP confers any long-term benefit it is probably by reducing the risk of oxygen toxicity by allowing the Fio_2 to be reduced below that which is necessary without PEEP. Although there are still arguments about the relevance of oxygen toxicity in the patient with lung damage, superoxide radicals can cause a type of alveolar damage which is very similar to ARDS. It is therefore advisable to use the lowest Fio_2 which, with the addition of minimal PEEP, will achieve a tolerable Pao_2. The safe/unsafe Fio_2 is not known with certainty but most clinicians would accept that the application of an Fio_2 of greater that 70% for more than a few hours is undesirable. If the arterial oxygen tension (Pao_2) is greater than 7.5 kPa no additional oxygen is required unless the patient has a high pyrexia or is hypercatabolic, in which case the lowest acceptable level is probably 8.0 kPa.

Unfortunately there is no evidence that the long-term survival of patients with established ARDS is improved when PEEP is used, although it is possible that death is postponed for a few days.

Extracorporeal Membrane Oxygenation (ECMO)

The use of this technique during open heart surgery led to the belief that its prolonged use could be of benefit for patients with potentially reversible lung lesions such as ARDS. Although anecdotal reports of its early use supported this belief, the controlled trial which was carried out under the auspices of the American National Heart and Lung Institute did not confirm these impressions, and with techniques at present available it should not be used.

An interesting variant of ECMO in which low frequency ventilation is combined with the extracorporeal removal of carbon dioxide has had some strikingly good results. This technique is under review at the present time.

DISSEMINATED INTRAVASCULAR COAGULATION

Many patients with ARDS have abnormal levels of coagulation factors. Thrombocytopenia is the most common isolated finding, and it if persists it has a bad prognostic significance, but rarely all of the signs of disseminated intravascular coagulation (DIC) may be recognized. The haematological criteria for making this diagnosis are not universally agreed but the following values are generally accepted:

1   Platelet count less than 60 000/cuml (normal range $200-500 \times 10^9/l$)
2   Fibrinogen level less than 1 g/l (normal range 2.5–4.0 g/l)
3   Prothrombin time less than 50% of normal (normal value 80%)
4   Fibrin degradation products more than 100 μg/ml (normal value 0–10 μg/ml)

It is a good policy not to treat the results of laboratory investigation but to treat the patient. Nevertheless, if these criteria are met and the patient shows evidence of bleeding from surgical wounds into the skin or elsewhere, or organ dysfunction—particularly respiratory or renal failure—heparinization may be necessary. Experimentally, the infusion of fibrin degradation products can increase vascular permeability which suggests that DIC may cause ARDS both by microembolism and by increasing capillary transudation.

Heparin should be given by infusion at 1000 u/h and its effects monitored with a device such as the 'Haemochron', which measures the activated clotting time. The objectives of treatment are to extend the clotting time by 25–30% whilst at the same time the platelet count should rise by at least $25 \times 10^9/l/24$ h.

Treatment with heparin in patients who have recently suffered major trauma or surgery is fraught with the risk of haemorrhage. In addition, even when tracheobronchial toilet is carried out with extreme care there is a constant risk of provoking intrapulmonary bleeding. 'Aeroflo' suction catheters or similar devices should be used when patients are heparinized or have other reasons for a tendency to bleed after minor trauma.

Miscellaneous aids to treatment

Ibuprofen, dazoxibenz and other prostaglandin inhibitors have been used in specialist centres both prophylactically and to treat the established disease. It is too early to be able to give an opinion as to their value. They have few side-effects and on theoretical grounds should be beneficial.

Experimentally, corticosteroids have been shown to reduce platelet aggregation. They have also been used for many years to treat pulmonary fibrosis. However, they have not reduced the mortality rate of ARDS and they also increase the risk of systemic sepsis and fluid retention; they should therefore not be used. Fibroblast infiltration and pulmonary fibrosis are prominent features of ARDS and substances are available which inhibit collagen synthesis; L-3,4-dehydroxyproline is the best known member of this group of drugs.

Unfortunately, none of these agents has been shown to influence the progress of ARDS. If a patient has florid DIC, heparinization may be indicated, but at the present time the value of the other agents is best assessed in those units which are equipped for research. Their more general use would inevitably lead to dissemination of anecdotal reports of success and/or failure which would not help the investigator, therapist or patient.

Avoidance of overload

This was emphasized earlier but repetition can only be beneficial. If, in addition to the signs of ARDS, the patient develops acute renal failure, it is essential to maintain immaculate fluid balance and to monitor the patient's intravascular volume. Central venous pressure monitoring may provide an early indication of right ventricular failure, although it is of limited value once the syndrome is established.

Normally the CVP rises when IPPV is applied; this is particularly noticeable when PEEP is used. Patients with ARDS have a markedly reduced pulmonary compliance and the CVP response to changes in intrathoracic pressure is very slow. If no CVP response occurs at all when IPPV is started or stopped the patient's prognosis is very poor.

Selection of infusion fluids

An attempt should be made to maintain the plasma oncotic pressure within normal limits by giving a balanced infusion regime which includes plasma proteins. This may not be entirely beneficial, since by giving radio-iodinated albumin it can be shown that some of the infused material quickly transudes into the alveoli, which may add to the difficulty of gaseous diffusion. The effective plasma oncotic pressure can now be measured at the bedside with a colloid osmometer.

It may be necessary to give repeated blood transfusions in order to maintain the patient's haemoglobin level at 10 g/dl which combines optimum oxygen carriage with optimum perfusion characteristics.

HYDROGEN ION DISTURBANCES AND THEIR CORRECTION

This topic is discussed in other texts, some of which are referred to at the end of this chapter, and only an outline can be given here.

When ARDS presents, the patient usually has a mixed respiratory and non-respiratory (metabolic) alkalaemia. A variety of factors is involved; these include hyperventilation and the metabolism of citrate from transfused blood. The intravenous administration of sodium bicarbonate during resuscitation may also contribute. During the later phase of the illness the patient often develops a non-respiratory acidaemia which may become severe enough to require correction. Although this is usually due to early renal failure, occasionally it is caused by lactic acid accumulation, and if the pH falls below 7.25 and the plasma lactate exceeds 10 mmol/l the patient's prognosis is poor. This is not specifically related to the plasma lactate level, but lactic acid accumulation indicates that the liver, kidneys and muscles are undergoing anaerobic metabolism which demonstrates the severity of the underlying systemic disturbance.

Correction of a base deficit

If the pH is below 7.30 and the base deficit exceeds -10 mmol/l corrective action should be taken. The extracellular fluid (ECF) volume is approximately 30% of the patient's body weight and the base excess (or deficit) is an indication of the buffering capacity of the ECF. The amount of sodium bicarbonate which is required to correct such a deficit is calculated from the equation:

$$\text{Base deficit} \times \frac{\text{Body weight (kg)}}{3} \times \text{mmol sodium bicarbonate}$$

Initially it is advisable to aim for partial correction: in other words, if the calculation suggests that 200 mmol sodium bicarbonate are required, only 100 mmol should be given and the blood gas analysis repeated after two hours. Further correction may then be given. Caution is recommended because large volumes of sodium bicarbonate may cause acute pulmonary oedema. In addition, since sodium bicarbonate does not cross cell membranes readily, an acute ionic disequilibrium may be caused, resulting in heart failure, coma and epileptiform convulsions. Acute changes in hydrogen ion status shift the position of the oxyhaemoglobin dissociation curve and interface with oxygen delivery to the tissues.

Haemodialysis

Many patients with ARDS show signs of renal impairment at some stage in their illness. These are described on p. 18, and it is the author's opinion that haemodialysis (or peritoneal dialysis) should be started early rather than waiting for the florid signs—which all too often include pulmonary oedema—to appear.

Once haemodialysis is established, the maintenance of zero fluid balance and correction of electrolyte disturbances is simplified and it also allows the patient to be given the requisite amount of calories and amino acids. The patient should be nursed on a weighing bed to allow changes in body weight to be recognized.

The use of catecholamines

The use of natural and synthetic catecholamines is described in Chapter 2. Many studies have shown that ARDS is associated with pulmonary hypertension, and the causative factors include alpha-adrenergic stimulation. Both isoprenaline and dobutamine improve pulmonary blood flow and reduce right ventricular end-diastolic pressure, although they may also increase $\dot{V}/Q$ imbalance and widen the Aa gradient. If either drug is used its effects must be monitored by frequent blood gas analysis, CVP and pulmonary wedge pressure measurement.

SUMMARY

ARDS is a complex condition which has its most obvious effects upon pulmonary gas exchange, but which involves every other organ and tissue. It has a high mortality rate which has not been reduced significantly by modern methods of treatment. Treatment should therefore be uncomplicated, atraumatic and non-invasive. Controlled ventilation with minimal oxygen and best PEEP, the avoidance of fluid overload, and the prevention of secondary infection are the cornerstones of treatment.

References

Ashbaugh, D.G., Bigelow, D.B., Petty, T.L & Levine, B.E. (1967) Acute respiratory distress in adults. *Lancet*, **ii**, 319–323.
Butler, W.J., Bohn, D.J., Bryan, A.C. & Froese, A.B. (1980) Ventilation by high frequency oscillation in humans. *Anesthesia and Analgesia*, **59**(8), 577–584.

Colman, R.W., Robboy, S.J. & Minna, J.D. (1972) Disseminated intravascular coagulation—an approach. *Journal of the American Medical Association*, **52**, 679–683.

Fein, A.M., Goldberg, S.K., Lippman, M.L. et al (1982) Adult respiratory distress syndrome. *British Journal of Anaesthesia*, **54**, 723–735.

Hardaway, R.M. (1973) Disseminated intravascular coagulation as a possible cause of acute respiratory failure. *Surgery, Gynecology and Obstetrics*, **137**, 1–5.

Malik, A.B. & Newell, J.C. (1977) Pulmonary perfusion and gas exchange in hemorrhage and shock. *Journal of Applied Physiology: Respiratory, Environmental and Exercise Physiology*, **42**(2), 279–286.

National Heart, Lung and Blood Institute: Division of Lung Diseases (1979) *Extracorporeal Support for Respiratory Insufficiency*. 243–245. Bethesda, Maryland: National Institutes of Health.

Parratt, J.R. & Sturgess, R.M. (1977) The possible roles of histamine, 5-hydroxytryptamine and prostaglandin F_2 alpha as mediators of the acute pulmonary effects of endotoxin. *British Journal of Pharmacology*, **60**, 209–219.

Rinaldo, J.E. & Roger, R.M. (1982) Adult respiratory distress syndrome; changing concepts of lung injury and repair. *New England Journal of Medicine*, **306**, 900–909.

Rizk, N.W. & Murray, J.F. (1982) PEEP and pulmonary edema. *American Journal of Medicine*, **72**, 381–383.

Saldeen, T. (1976) The microembolism syndrome. *Microvascular Research*, **11**, 227–259.

Shoemaker, W.C. (1976) *The Lung in the Critically Ill Patient*. 127 pp. Baltimore: Williams and Wilkins.

Sibbald, W.J., Anderson, R.R. & Holliday, R.L. (1979) Pathogenesis of pulmonary oedema associated with the adult respiratory distress syndrome. *Canadian Medical Association Journal*, **120**, 445–450.

Staub, N.C. (1971) Steady state transvascular water filtration in unanesthetized sheep. *Circulation Research*, **28** Suppl. 1, 135–139.

Stoddart, J.C. (1982) Hydrogen ion regulation. In *Metabolic Care* (Ed.) Tweedle, D.E.F. Chapter 4. Edinburgh and London: Churchill Livingstone.

Suter, P.M., Fairley, H.B. & Isenberg, B.D. (1975) Optimum end expiratory airway pressure in patients with acute pulmonary failure. *New England Journal of Medicine*, **291**, 284–289.

Tillo, G.B., Johnson, H.J., Hunkel, R. & Ward, P.A. (1982) Intravascular activation of complement and acute lung injury. Dependency on neutrophils and toxic oxygen metabolites. *Journal of Clinical Investigation*, **69**, 1126–1135.

Traber, D.L., Adams, T., Henriksen, N. & Traber, R.N. (1981) Ibuprofen and diphenhydramine protect the lung in sepsis. *Anesthesiology*, **55**(3) ASA Abstract A76.

Zapol, W.M. & Sinden, M.T. (1977) Pulmonary hypertension in severe acute pulmonary failure. *New England Journal of Medicine*, **296**, 476–480.

6

Fat Embolism and the Fat Embolism Syndrome

The subject discussed in this chapter shares many features with the adult respiratory distress syndrome, but its onset is usually more easily recognized, its cause relatively well understood and its prognosis much better.

The distinction between fat embolism and the fat embolism syndrome should be recognized at the outset. Up to 90% of patients who have suffered major trauma which includes bone injury can be shown at autopsy to have fat droplet deposits in the lungs and elsewhere, without necessarily having shown any evidence of this phenomenon in life. The fat embolism syndrome is much less common but it may present a threat to the patient's survival and always gives rise to identifiable symptoms.

DEFINITION OF THE FAT EMBOLISM SYNDROME

The syndrome may be defined as a condition which is usually associated with long bone fractures, with symptoms attributable to obstruction of the small blood vessels of many organs and tissues. Very occasionally the fat embolism syndrome has been described after trauma to adipose tissue, to the liver, the spleen and the pancreas, but in these instances it is probably more appropriate to group the cause in the ARDS/DIC category. This point will be emphasized later.

The distinction between fat embolism and the fat embolism syndrome is thought to be due to the total mass of fat which is released into the circulation from the traumatized tissues. It is believed that the fat droplets must exceed $8\,\mu$ in diameter before they can give rise to symptoms. The emboli are thought to block small arterioles and capillaries, after which they are coated with platelets. Plasma lipase converts the neutral fat to free fatty acids which damage the alveolar capillary cells and, together with lysed platelets, gives rise to the sequence of events described in the last chapter with release of thromboxane, prostaglandin F_2 alpha, 5-hydroxytryptamine, and histamine.

Alternative sources of fat emboli

Some investigators believe that the fat emboli do not necessarily originate from bone marrow but may be formed by the coalescence of fat chylomicrons, which are normally less than $1\,\mu$ in diameter, through the increased secretion of corticosteroids and catecholamines which follows trauma. It is known that catecholamines can increase the level of circulating lipids which are then converted to fatty acids. The fat embolism syndrome has been diagnosed following the use of high dose corticosteroids, but since these drugs are commonly given to patients who are suffering from acute cardiocirculatory failure due to trauma or sepsis, the relevance of these reports is questionable. ARDS is indistinguishable from the respiratory effects of fat embolism.

It is generally accepted that fat emboli contain mostly triglyceride fat, whereas coalesced chylomicrons or fat from adipose tissue should contain cholesterol; this has only rarely been identified in embolic material. Occasionally bone marrow cells and even spicules of bone have been identified in embolic material found in the lungs and elsewhere of patients who have died following injuries to the bony skeleton.

Many attempts have been made to identify pathological quantities of fat and fat droplets in the plasma of patients suffering from the fat embolism syndrome, but these have not been generally successful.

Whatever the origin of the fat may be, pathologists agree that if the patient survives for seven days or more after the event, no fat emboli can be identified in the lungs or elsewhere, although stigmata of their recent presence may be found. These include small haemosiderin deposits surrounding cerebral arterioles and areas of microinfarction in the renal cortex. The respiratory evidence is usually obscured by the tissue reaction which is typical of ARDS.

CLINICAL FEATURES OF THE FAT EMBOLISM SYNDROME

Classically these appear within 72 hours of a fracture of a long bone such as the femur or tibia. Other bony injuries (ribs, sternum, pelvis) may also provoke this reaction, and it may follow orthopaedic manoeuvres. The syndrome which occasionally follows the impaction of methyl methacrylate cement into the bone marrow is almost certainly identical. One of the most interesting aspects of the fat embolism syndrome is that it has never been known to develop twice in the same patient in spite of repeated orthopaedic manipulations of the original injury.

Presentation

Breathlessness, confusion, restlessness or coma are the most common presenting features, and grand mal seizures may occur. The patient usually has an irritating cough, with or without haemoptysis. Occasionally it may present as failure to regain consciousness following orthopaedic manipulations performed under general anaesthesia. Focal neurological signs such as hemiplegia or paraplegia may appear but are unusual and should cause the attendant to consider the possibility of more extensive intracranial damage. This should always be excluded before the treatment regimen described later is instituted, and computerized axial tomography (CAT scan) may be necessary. The possibility of intracranial damage must always be considered if the patient has a history of transient loss of consciousness at the time of the injury or shortly afterwards.

Although frank haematuria may be noted, this is unusual, but most patients with fat embolism syndrome have microscopic haematuria.

Pathophysiology

How embolic material which is small enough to pass through the pulmonary capillaries can obstruct the cerebral and renal vasculature is still debated, but three explanations have been propounded. Twenty-five per cent of all patients who are submitted to autopsy examination are found to have a potentially patent foramen ovale. This would permit a right-to-left shunt to develop in the presence of the pulmonary hypertension which follows extensive pulmonary fat embolism. Pulmonary arteriovenous shunts have been identified and these also present a pathway for embolic material. Disseminated intravascular coagulation, possibly activated by the circulating free fatty acids, is the third possible mechanism although the laboratory signs of DIC are only rarely identified.

Blood gas effects

If the patient's blood gases are measured at this stage a variable degree of hypoxia is always recognizable, and many authorities state categorically that the neurological effects of fat embolism are due to cerebral hypoxia. This is not so; the author has treated many patients with fat embolism in whom the level of oxygen desaturation is not severe enough to explain the neurological symptoms. For example, a young patient with normal blood vessels does not become confused or comatose with a Pao_2 of 7.0 kPa or more. On the other hand, if the patient is very hypoxic he may present with diffuse neurological symptoms, of which confusion is the commonest, and which may improve when he is given oxygen-enriched air to breath. Cerebral fat embolism may cause confusion in the absence of systemic hypoxia and vice versa. The early development of neurological signs distinguishes fat embolism syndrome from ARDS.

The respiratory and neurological features of the syndrome often appear concurrently but may be discrete. Dyspnoea, tachypnoea, bronchospasm and pulmonary oedema may occur separately or together. These symptoms are often mistaken for bronchopneumonia, particularly since the patient may also have an elevated temperature. At this stage, a chest radiograph shows the typical 'snow storm' appearance but later the lung fields may be diffusely radio-opaque.

Skin manifestations

A petechial rash is the third feature of the syndrome, although this often appears without any systemic symptoms or signs. It is usually most noticeable on the anterior axillary folds, in the base of the neck and close to the inguinal ligaments, but it may become generalized and successive showers of petechiae may be recognised. The spots may also be noted in the lower conjunctival sac and, if the fundi are examined during the early phase, fat droplets are occasionally seen passing through the retinal veins. The petechiae are 1–3 mm in diameter and initially are red but quickly turn brown. If a skin biopsy is taken fat droplets can be seen in the dermal capillaries. Fat droplets may occasionally be identified in sputum and in urine but these are not diagnostic features of the syndrome since both false-positive and false-negative findings are common.

Stress peptic ulcer

Patients with the fat embolism syndrome are said to be at special risk of stress peptic ulceration. This has been attributed to mucosal infarction, but in the injured patient all of the standard causes of stress ulceration are present and it has been suggested that hypothalamic fat can increase gastric acid secretion.

Haematological features

Up to 50% of patients with fat embolism develop thrombocytopenia, and hypocalcaemia is also common. This latter finding is said to be due to the affinity for calcium ions of the free fatty acids released as the emboli are hydrolysed. The haemoglobin level may fall as much as 3 g/dl in 48 hours without obvious cause, although continued bleeding around closed fractures, into the gastrointestinal tract or other occult sites is the more likely explanation. Usually, thrombocytopenia is an isolated finding, but occasionally all of the laboratory features of DIC are noted, together with its clinical signs. At this stage the syndrome blends into DIC/ARDS, with its additional problems.

Patients with multiple injuries may develop fat embolism, with or without the 'syndrome'; they may develop ARDS without petechiae or cerebral signs of fat embolism; they may present with bleeding due to DIC with the involvement of the other organs being noted only secondarily.

The relationship between fat embolism and DIC is at present a matter for speculation since fat droplets per se do not activate the coagulation cascade. If the emboli impact and cause extensive tissue damage, DIC could be provoked, but this degree of infarction is unusual. It is probable that the mechanisms which provoke fat embolism and DIC occur in parallel rather than being directly related, that is, they are separate manifestations of acute traumatic cardiocirculatory failure.

CLINICAL COURSE OF THE FAT EMBOLISM SYNDROME

The severity of the illness is largely related to the extent of the injuries, and after very extensive fractures patients may succumb within 24 hours of the incident from diffuse embolic disease. However, trivial injuries may occasionally cause death from fat embolism. Some procedures have an ominous reputation; this is particularly the case with the open reduction and nailing of sub-capital femoral neck fractures.

Prognosis of fat embolism

The most challenging feature of the condition is its unpredictable nature, and the mortality rates quoted by different authorities range from 5 to 15%. A patient who presents with a florid rash, cyanosed, breathless and with a tachydysrhythmia may either improve steadily with only minimal treatment, or progress inexorably downhill with a widening Aa gradient and die days later from intractable hypoxia with evidence of multiple organ involvement.

The neurological effects of fat embolism have a good prognosis for functional recovery, provided that the patient's respiratory dysfunction is reversible. Patients who die in the acute phase of the disease are usually found to have many hundreds of petechial haemorrhages scattered throughout the cerebral white and grey matter and the basal nuclei. If the patient survives the immediate insult but dies days or weeks later, no gross areas of cerebral infarction are found. Patients who develop paraplegia or other focal signs have a less predictable prognosis.

TREATMENT OF THE FAT EMBOLISM SYNDROME

Hypoxia is the most dangerous feature of this condition and, ideally, every patient with long bone injuries should have his PaO_2 measured at least once each day for the first five days after the injury. Unfortunately, blood gas analysis is not routinely performed in most orthopaedic wards, and in many cases hypoxia is not recognized until it is clinically obvious, by which time the patient is usually very ill.

As soon as the diagnosis is made the patient should be given 100% oxygen by face mask and the arterial oxygen tension monitored. Preferably he should be admitted to the ITU immediately because he may deteriorate rapidly and require controlled ventilation with added oxygen. Baseline data should be obtained to identify the involvement of other organs, and a comprehensive neurological examination must be performed.

Pulmonary hypertension and pulmonary oedema

Pulmonary hypertension is an early manifestation of pulmonary fat embolism. This can be recognized clinically by auscultation when the second pulmonary sound is noted to be accentuated, or by means of a Swan Ganz catheter. Most patients have clinical and radiographic evidence of pulmonary oedema. Although this is usually due to the fat and its breakdown products, over-enthusiastic intravenous fluid administration may also be involved. In either case, when the diagnosis is made the patient should be given frusemide 20–40 mg intravenously and his arterial oxygen tension and Aa gradient measured after the subsequent diuresis. If these improve it may be advisable to give a second dose of frusemide. Every patient with the fat embolism syndrome should be maintained in perfect fluid balance until he has recovered.

Respiratory care

If oxygen by mask does not have the desired result, the patient should be sedated, intubated and ventilated; this may be required because the patient is exhausted by tachypnoea. IPPV may be required for up to ten days, but unless the patient develops a chest infection tracheostomy should not be necessary since in many cases recovery is rapid and uncomplicated. However, if the Pao_2 continues to fall in spite of increasing the Pio_2 and adding PEEP, the prognosis is poor.

Other aids to treatment

The following list includes most of the agents which have been used to treat fat embolism.
1   Heparin—to speed lipolysis and reduce platelet adhesiveness.
2   Alcohol—to dissolve fat and act as a vasodilator.
3   Aprotinin—to inhibit protein breakdown in embolized pulmonary capillaries.
4   Corticosteroids—to reduce leucocyte aggregation, preserve lysosomal membranes, and prevent the formation of vasodepressor kinins.
5   Dextran 40—to improve capillary flow.
6   Clofibrate—to reduce plasma lipids.
7   Acetyl salicylic acid—to reduce platelet adhesiveness.
8   Prostacyclin—to reduce platelet adhesiveness.

None of these agents has been shown to produce any clear-cut improvement, and some may be positively harmful. Heparin may aggravate the syndrome by encouraging the breakdown of triclyceride fat to fatty acids which provoke a more violent tissue response. Dextran 40 is contraindicated in the presence of renal impairment. Corticosteroids belong to the ever increasing number of drugs whose actions consist almost entirely of side-effects; these include the encouragement of sepsis, pulmonary oedema and peptic ulceration. None of the published papers which attribute success to their use has demonstrated statistically significant improvement.

If the patient develops fulminant DIC, heparinization may be necessary. Since DIC does not usually develop until two to three days after the initial symptoms, most of the fat emboli will have lysed by this stage, and heparin may not be harmful. However, the prognosis for a patient with this combination of symptoms is uniformly bad.

The prognosis for patients with fat embolism syndrome is very unpredictable. Treatment should be based upon fundamental principles which include maintenance of gas exchange, prevention or treatment of fluid overload and pulmonary oedema, and the avoidance of potentially harmful agents.

PREVENTION OF FAT EMBOLISM

In the present state of knowledge this desirable aim appears to be unattainable. Most orthopaedic surgeons believe that fracture manipulations should be applied as gently as possible, as late as possible, but there is still no substitute for careful monitoring and early treatment. Delayed recognition of fat embolism syndrome allows the complications of coma and infection to be added to what is still a dangerous condition.

SUMMARY

Fat embolism and the fat embolism syndrome are conditions in which fat droplets are released into the circulation from bone marrow after trauma; rarely the syndrome may follow soft tissue injuries. If the droplets are large enough they may lodge in the capillaries and larger vessels of the skin, brain, lung and elsewhere. In most cases the condition is self-limiting. Treatment should be aimed at providing support for vital organs, using techniques which are as simple and innocuous as possible, until recovery occurs.

References

Bergentz, S.E. (1968) Fat embolism. *Progress in Surgery*, **6,** 85–120.

Cole, W.G. (1971) Clofibrate and fat embolism. *British Medical Journal*, **2,** 148–149.

Gardner, A.M.N. & Harrison, C.M.H.M. (1957) The treatment of experimental fat embolism with heparin. *Journal of Bone and Joint Surgery*, **39B,** 538–540.

Gossling, H.R. & Pellegrini, V.D. (1982) Fat embolism syndrome. *Clinical Orthopaedics and Related Research*, **165**(5)**,** 68–82.

Gurd, A.R. (1970) Fat embolism; an aid to diagnosis. *Journal of Bone and Joint Surgery*, **52B,** 732–737.

Herndon, J.H., Riseborough, E.J. & Fischer J.E. (1971) Fat embolism; a review of current concepts. *Journal of Trauma,* **11**(8)**,** 673–680.

Lessells, A.M. (1981) Fatal fat embolism after minor trauma. *British Medical Journal*, **1,** 1586.

Sevitt, S. (1962) *Fat Embolism.* 233 pp. London: Butterworths.

Szabo, G. (1970) The syndrome of fat embolism and its origin. *Journal of Clinical Pathology*, Supplement 4, 123–131.

Watson, A.J. (1970) Genesis of fat embolism. *Journal of Clinical Pathology,* Supplement 4, 132–142.

7

Burns and Inhalation Damage

L. J. DUNKIN

Epidemiology and mortality

Approximately 70% of patients with burns who are admitted to hospital receive their injuries in the home. Scalding and clothing fires are more common in children, whilst bedding and house fires are most likely to affect the elderly and infirm. Industrial accidents account for about 25% of burns admissions and occur within the age range of the working population.

The mortality rate is closely related to the percentage burn surface area (BSA) and the age of the victim, there being a reduced survival rate for patients at the lower and upper end of the age spectrum. A multifactorial probit analysis has shown that the area of full thickness burns, previous bronchopulmonary disease, arterial oxygen tension on admission and the presence of airway oedema are other decisive factors.

Burns units

The development of burns units after World War II increased the overall survival rate from thermal injury and also improved function and cosmetic results; patients with burns of 25% BSA or over should, if possible, be transferred to such a unit as soon as immediate care has been started. Less extensive burns involving the face, hands, feet and genitalia or patients with respiratory damage need treatment in the best available centre. Children also benefit from specialized care, preferably in burns units. All Accident Departments should have information packs available which contain tables, charts and action cards outlining the essential care requirements of all age groups.

The burns team

Trauma services and plastic surgery departments usually bear immediate responsibility for the treatment of burns, but clinical physiologists, renal physicians, nutritionists and microbiologists also play a role. Anaesthetists who have a special interest in resuscitation, respiratory support and intensive care can also contribute, in addition to providing anaesthesia and analgesia.

Much of the day-to-day treatment is provided by the nursing staff who make a major contribution to the work of the team. Good functional recovery requires early attention to positioning, exercises and splinting; this is the province of the physiotherapy staff who also assist with the care of patients who develop pulmonary problems.

Surface burns

The skin is the largest organ system of the body and has a surface area of 1.5–2 m^2 in the adult. It fulfils many important functions, and the destruction or damage of a significant area of skin has serious consequences. The depth of burn is the major factor in determining the outcome. The long-established classification into first, second or third degree burns has been simplified into:

Partial thickness—superficial or deep;
Full thickness.

The physiological sequelae of serious skin burns extend over a number of weeks. The effects follow a predictable triphasic pattern:

Phase I—capillary leakage, hypovolaemia, hypoxia, oliguria.
Phase II—capillary recovery, normovolaemia, anaemia.
Phase III—hypermetabolism, exudation, diuresis, dehydration, infection, anaemia.

These phases are not necessarily separate but often overlap. They do however indicate the general progression of events to be expected and treated following burn injury. Complications may arise during any phase, further affecting progress and prognosis.

PHASE I

Pathophysiology

Circulation

Depending upon the temperature and duration of exposure, heat destroys superficial capillaries and damages those lying deeper. The permeability of the latter is increased by the injury and by the release of histamine and other vasoactive mediators. These agents also cause temporary arteriolar dilatation, which raises the hydrostatic pressure within the capillaries and augments the loss of protein-rich fluid into the surrounding tissues.

In a major burn the consequent reduction in plasma volume has two critical effects, namely hypovolaemia and increased viscosity from haemoconcentration. Both of these phenomena result in diminished cardiac output and tissue perfusion leading to hypoxia and major organ dysfunction. It has also been demonstrated that heart muscle can be damaged by a specific cardiac depressant factor produced from major burns, further reducing circulatory efficiency.

Considerable numbers of red cells are destroyed by direct heat or by lysing factors produced from damaged tissue. The resulting loss of red cell mass is masked by the initial haemoconcentration, but haemoglobinuria provides evidence of the underlying erythrocyte disruption. There is, in addition, a degree of red cell distortion which further alters capillary flow and oxygen flux in the tissues. Oxygen availability is reduced with consequent acidosis. The sodium pump may be damaged, allowing sodium to accumulate within the cell. This may be a key factor in burn shock, and an average adult with 40% burns may require up to 1400 mmol of sodium to maintain normal extracellular levels in the first 24 hours.

Following circumferential burns limb viability may be threatened if the contraction of deeply damaged skin acts as a tourniquet, cutting off the arterial supply. In addition, unsuspected oedema within the deeper myofascial compartments may result in compression and ischaemic contractures.

Respiratory system

Arterial hypoxaemia is a common finding in severe burns, even in the absence of inhalation damage. Postmortem studies in fatal cases may reveal changes ranging from a moderate increase in lung water to frank adult respiratory distress syndrome. In experimental animals with 50% skin burns there was a reduced ventilation–perfusion ratio and a low Pao_2 associated with complement activation, leucocyte aggregation and capillary microthrombi. Inhalation damage and infection may further complicate the pulmonary changes, as will be described later.

Hyperventilation is common and may be due in part to the low Pao_2 or to elevated circulating catecholamine levels. The topical dressing 'mafenide' may also cause hyperventilation. In contrast, patients with over 40% BSA involving the trunk have been found to have a mild to moderate restrictive disorder characterized by a reduction in vital capacity. Although chest wall damage may play a part, other factors are involved. Circumferential full thickness burns of the thorax will have a restrictive effect needing urgent escharotomy. Deep burns of the neck following electrical injury may cause temporary phrenic nerve paralysis.

Renal function

Patients with severe burns frequently develop acute renal failure. The causes include those discussed in Chapter 2, but it is possible that myoglobin and haemoglobin from charred tissue and red cells play a particularly important part. Vascular access for haemodialysis may present a difficult problem, and peritoneal dialysis may have to be performed through burned abdominal skin and subcutaneous tissues.

Treatment of Phase I

This section describes the treatment which is required during the first 36–48 hours following the injury. Not all burns will require the full regimen and, where appropriate, treatment may be adjusted to suit patients with less extensive skin damage. Those with less than 15% BSA can usually tolerate oral fluid replacement. In other cases oral intake may supplement intravenous fluid if gastrointestinal function is satisfactory.

Some patients with severe burns seem reasonably well when first seen but the loss of fluid into the tissues has already begun and must be treated. Others may, on admission, exhibit the full picture of burn shock including peripheral circulatory failure with cold extremities, cyanosis, tachycardia, low BP, restlessness and thirst. The presence of facial burns should lead to suspicion of inhalation damage causing progressive airway obstruction and possibly lung dysfunction. In this critical situation it is essential to have an agreed plan of action for immediate implementation.

Immediate care

1 Airway patency and breathing must be quickly checked and 50% oxygen given by mask. Should it be necessary, the patient is intubated.
2 Using the Rules of Nine method (Figure 17) a rapid examination is carried out to assess the approximate BSA, excluding unblistered erythematous areas. Where it exceeds 15% in adults (10% in children) intravenous resuscitation is necessary.
3 A wide-bore free-flowing cannula is inserted in the largest available vein using a cut-down through burned skin if necessary. At the same time a sample of venous blood is taken for haematology, electrolytes, carboxyhaemoglobin and grouping.
4 Depending upon unit policy, an infusion of plasma protein fraction (PPF) or Ringers lactate is started and a rapid estimate is made of fluid needs in the first few hours from one of the formulae on page 111.
5 Pain may be severe and where there are no respiratory contraindications 2 mg increments of papaveretum are given intravenously up to a total of 15 mg over ten minutes, the effect of each increment being carefully assessed before proceeding. Full thickness areas are pain-free, and where these predominate analgesia requirements may be less.

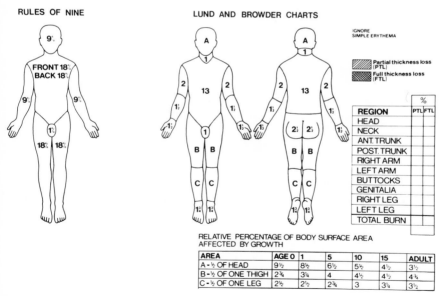

RELATIVE PERCENTAGE OF BODY SURFACE AREA AFFECTED BY GROWTH

AREA	AGE 0	1	5	10	15	ADULT
A - ½ OF HEAD	9½	8½	6½	5½	4½	3½
B - ½ OF ONE THIGH	2¾	3¼	4	4½	4½	4¾
C - ½ OF ONE LEG	2½	2½	2¾	3	3¼	3½

Figure 17. The Rules of Nine (left) and the Lund and Browder (right) methods of assessing burn surface area.

6   If not already in the burns unit the patient should now be transferred there and full monitoring of all vital signs begun.

7   A central line, nasogastric tube and urinary catheter are inserted aseptically and gently and a full examination is carried out to exclude any other injuries. If facial burns are present the eyes should be examined before oedema closes the lids.

8   A chest radiograph should be taken to check the lung fields and establish the position of the central line and nasogastric tube.

9   An antacid (such as magnesium trisilicate) is given down the nasogastric tube and ranitidine injected intravenously.

10   An arterial blood sample is taken for blood gas analysis.

11   If the patient has limb burns, a regular check on peripheral pulses is begun and charted.

12   Before the application of dressings the original calculation of BSA should be rechecked using the more precise method of Lund and Browder (Figure 17) and to the burn depth reassessed.

13   Blisters which interfere with function are removed and the burns dressed.

Treatment of hypovolaemia

Choice of resuscitation fluid

A decision has to be made as to the type of fluid to use: crystalloid, colloid, or a mixture of both. The colloid used is usually plasma protein fraction (PPF) although other volume expanders have been employed.

Since much of the infused fluid is lost into the tissues in the early stages of resuscitation it would seem reasonable to conserve expensive and scarce supplies of plasma. Furthermore, reabsorption of oedema fluid may be more rapid if it contains less protein. However, it has been shown in thermally injured animals that fluid lost from the intravascular compartment is inversely proportional to the albumin content in the infusion fluid. Burn oedema is not necessarily confined to the burn area, and an increased water content in the lungs is more likely after crystalloid resuscitation than when colloid is used.

When only minimal amounts of PPF have been given the serum protein level must be measured after 48 hours and any deficiency rectified. On the other hand if a 'plasma only' regimen is pursued it is important to ensure that the ionized calcium level is adequate, and if necessary calcium chloride supplements can be given. Whatever type of infusion fluid is employed it is essential to restore depleted extracellular sodium levels, although the sick cell syndrome should be borne in mind, and sodium overload avoided. PPF contains 140–160 mmol/l of sodium and Ringer's lactate 131 mmol/l sodium.

Assessment of intravenous volume requirements

The rate of fluid loss from the circulation cannot be determined accurately in the early stages. Adjustments may be needed during the progress of resuscitation. Depending largely on the type of fluid employed the formulae aim to provide between 2 and 4 ml/kg/% BSA in the first 24 hours.

Two such formulae are described below: the modified Mount Vernon

Hospital Plan (I), which is widely used in the United Kingdom, and the formula based on that employed at the Brooke Army Hospital in Texas (II). For both formulae, unless it is known accurately, the patient's weight is estimated from the measured height and body build. All calculations are made from the actual time of the burn injury.

Formula I (Mount Vernon)

This uses plasma protein fraction (PPF) as volume replacement, and dextrose 5% to meet water needs. It was originally calculated for freeze-dried plasma, but with the introduction of PPF it has been found necessary to increase the volume by about one-third.

1 Divide the first 36 hours from the time of the burn into six periods of 4, 4, 4, 6, 6 and 12 hours.

2 In each period give plasma (PPF, Plasmanate):

$$\frac{BSA\% \times Wt \text{ in } kg \times 2}{3} \, ml$$

A convenient calculator has been described which quickly gives the correct volume of plasma for each period.

3 Over the full 36 hours give dextrose 5% in water: 40–50 ml/kg.

The dextrose in water should not be started until there is reasonable evidence that hypovolaemia is being corrected.

Formula II (Brooke Army Hospital)

Using the same basic data, including the time of the burn, this formula relies less heavily on plasma. The total quantity of fluid in the first 24 hours is calculated as follows:

1 Ringer's lactate: BSA% × Wt in kg × 1.5 ml.

2 Plasma (PPF, Plasmanate): BSA% × Wt in kg × 0.5 ml.

3 5% Dextrose in water: 2000 ml.

Half the total of (1) and (2) is given in the first eight hours and one-quarter in each of the two remaining eight-hour periods. As with Formula (I), the dextrose 5% is withheld until the initial oligaemia has been adequately corrected.

Although formulae provide a very useful guide some workers prefer to monitor haemodynamic variables and to administer fluid on an individualized basis.

Whole blood requirements

Where the full thickness burns area (FTBA) exceeds 15% of the body surface area, whole blood will be required to maintain red cell mass in the face of intravascular haemolysis. In the first 36 hours this may be estimated on the basis of one unit of blood for every 10% of FTBA.

Unless the FTBA exceeds 25% it may be best to delay transfusions until the haematocrit begins to fall. The blood should then be given instead of an equivalent volume of plasma. In the event of other injuries, such as open wounds or closed fractures, the amount and timing of blood transfusion may have to be altered. Where possible, recently donated blood should be used in order to achieve maximal red cell life in the recipient, who may have a raised level of plasma haemolysins.

Monitoring the burned patient

Patients who have suffered extensive burns require continuous and comprehensive monitoring as outlined on pages 25–26.

Inadequate response to volume replacement

Although most patients respond to the measures recommended above, signs of inadequate response include:
1   Central cyanosis and altered level of consciousness
2   Tachycardia with weak, thready pulse and low BP
3   Low CVP and PCWP
4   Urinary output less than 30 ml/h
5   Increased skin–core temperature difference

These signs are usually caused by hypovolaemia, and fluid resuscitation should be increased until a response is obtained. Where there is adequate volume loading but poor urinary output, dopamine may be given, as described on page 35. The further management of oliguria and renal failure is discussed on page 17.

Analgesia

Adequate analgesia is an important aspect of treatment when the pain of partial thickness burns is severe. Pain relief may be achieved by 15 mg papaveretum diluted in saline and given intravenously in 2 mg increments until an adequate level of analgesia is achieved. The respiratory rate and depth should be assessed before each increment is given; if there is any question of airway involvement oxygen and a means of hand ventilation must always be available. Analgesia may be maintained by a continuous infusion of papaveretum 2–5 mg per hour. The respiratory rate must not fall below 10 bpm and blood gas figures should be checked to ensure that ventilation is adequate. The infusions may be increased under direct medical supervision for carrying out painful procedures, such as burns dressings.

In the later management of pain, opiate analgesics may be given orally or sublingually, night sedation being added as required. It may also be necessary to employ medication to relieve anxiety or improve mood during a prolonged stay in hospital.

Environment

Although it is not possible to prevent bacterial contamination of burns, every effort must be made to reduce the occurrence of bacterial transfer within the burns unit. Each hospital should have a set of rules suited to its particular needs and these should be carefully observed by all members of the team.

It is helpful to place the extensively burned patient on some form of special support system such as the 'Clinitron' bead-bed. In this the patient, lying on a porous sheet, floats in a medium of siliconized glass microspheres which are fluidized by a continuous current of warm filtered air. It is comfortable for the patient and, when combined with a warm ambient temperature, assists in reducing heat loss which may be of considerable importance in the later hypermetabolic state.

Local treatment of burns

Topical applications

Most of the history of burns care has centred around different topical treatments. The Chinese employed tea extract (tannin) 70 centuries ago; Pliny the Elder recommended exposure to air, while in the seventh century AD Arabian physicians prescribed cold water to alleviate pain—all methods which were to find favour again many centuries later.

The development of topically applied chemotherapeutic preparations has brought about a considerable reduction in burn wound sepsis and related morbidity. They are applied liberally, as aseptically as possible, soon after admission and the wounds are then covered with absorbent dressings; these include mafenide and silver sulphadiazine creams. Mafenide has a wide spectrum of antibacterial activity but the 12-hourly applications are rather painful. In addition, as an inhibitor of carbonic anhydrase, it may lead to non-respiratory acidosis and cause compensatory hyperventilation. Silver sulphadiazine is also useful although it is not as penetrating as mafenide, and it may cause a mild leucopenia. It is however painless to apply. These preparations limit bacterial invasion in the earlier management, pending effective wound cover with skin or skin substitutes.

Escharotomy

Where full thickness circumferential burns occur the resulting thick and unyielding scar can have constricting effects and threaten blood supply to limbs or reduce chest expansion. Releasing incisions down to subcutaneous fat should be carried out with a minimum of delay. Since such skin is insensitive, general anaesthesia is not required. Fasciotomy may be necessary after very deep burns to decompress myofascial compartments but this will require general anaesthesia.

PHASE II

Pathophysiology

Within 24 hours of the injury the capillary bed begins to recover and becomes less permeable to plasma proteins. Lymphatic drainage and the gradual restoration of oncotic pressure gradients encourage re-entry of sequestrated fluid into the intravascular compartment and the re-establishment of normovolaemia. However, some local oedema is slow to clear due to a combination of residual capillary and lymphatic dysfunction. As internal restoration of plasma volume takes place, external fluid losses from the injured areas increase, reaching the very high levels described in Phase III.

Even when blood has been given during the first 36 hours, re-expansion of the plasma volume frequently reveals a red cell deficit. Lysing factors in the plasma shorten erythrocyte life-span; there is commonly a persistent anaemia despite apparently adequate blood transfusion.

Treatment of Phase II

During this brief period there is a change of emphasis from plasma volume restoration to the replenishment of evaporative water loss with 5% dextrose solution at a rate of about 1–2 ml/kg/%BSA/day. To this is added the normal daily water and electrolyte requirements. If the patient can drink or if a nasogastric tube is in situ and gut function has returned enteral fluids may be given. As the haemoglobin begins to fall blood transfusion may be necessary. If no blood has been transfused in the first 36 hours the formula given on page 111 may be used. Where a diuresis has not yet started and the central venous pressure is elevated it may be advisable to induce a diuresis with frusemide and to give packed cells to avoid circulatory overload, especially in elderly subjects.

PHASE III

Pathophysiology

Fluid and electrolyte changes

Following on the immediate post-burn sequence of oedema–hypovolaemia–volume replacement, patients should reach this phase in positive fluid balance. As the extravasated fluid re-enters the circulation and the secretion of ADH and aldosterone falls, the kidneys respond with a diuresis of water, sodium and potassium. At the same time increasing amounts of fluid are lost from the wound surface, both by evaporation and by exudation. The exudate has a high sodium content and losses are proportionate to the surface area of the burn. These losses may cause patients to swing from a positive to a negative water and electrolyte balance within a fairly short time-span.

Even when attempts are made to replace output on a quantitative basis, imbalances may occur and regular laboratory checks are necessary to watch for the opposing clinical phases of:
1 Dehydration–overload
2 Hyponatraemia—hypernatraemia
3 Hypokalaemia—hyperkalaemia
4 Acidosis—alkalosis

Metabolic changes

The endocrine response to burns injury includes a persistent catecholamine drive with an increase in glucocorticoid and glucagon levels. Insulin activity is suppressed, giving rise to the 'pseudo-diabetes' of thermal injury. During this phase there is also a dramatic rise in metabolic rate which, in burns of up to 50%, bears a linear relationship to the BSA. Hypermetabolism can be reduced by increasing the ambient temperature.

As a consequence of the hypermetabolic state there is an increased oxygen demand, at a time when oxygen uptake in the lung may be compromised for a number of reasons, including inhalation damage; in addition, anaemia will reduce the oxygen-carrying capacity of the blood. It is not surprising, therefore, that the cardiac output rises in figures considerably above normal to meet this oxygen need.

Enormous nitrogen losses occur in severely burned patients, partly due to leakage of protein-rich exudates from the burns wound, but mainly as a result of muscle proteolysis. The amino acids released by this process are converted into glucose within the liver and the nitrogen converted to urea for excretion by the kidney.

Liver and kidney function

Depending on the size of the burn and the degree of early tissue hypoxia, some hepatocellular damage is common, as is confirmed by liver function tests and, in those patients who do not survive, by the presence of histological changes. This is usually temporary but it may progress to liver failure as a result of toxaemia and infection, combined with excessive metabolic and excretory demands. The effect of burns and shock upon the kidney have already been referred to.

Infection

Probably one-third of the patients with over 30% burns who do not survive die from infection. Areas of necrotic tissue become contaminated with a wide variety of organisms which have changed over the years from gram-positive to gram-negative bacteria; anaerobes, yeasts, fungi and viruses are also involved. They cause further necrosis of underlying tissues, thus converting a partial thickness into a full thickness skin loss. The early use of topical chemotherapy reduces bacterial proliferation and this has reduced the morbidity and mortality resulting from infection.

Apart from the surface breach in the body's defences caused by the wound itself, there is a general reduction in the ability to respond to microbiological invasion. Neutrophil function is depressed and serum immunoglobulin levels are diminished at an early stage. The catabolic drive and nutritional problems cause subsequent difficulties in restoring normal immunocompetence. Thus when microbial invasion does occur, the full picture of toxaemia and septicaemia may finally progress to neutropenia, hypothermia and death.

Treatment of Phase III

Fluid and electrolyte replacement

The patient's intake must keep pace with the increasing losses. The daily requirement of water, sodium and potassium may be calculated as follows:
1 Urinary and other measurable loss of water and electrolytes.
2 Evaporation and fluid exudate from wound: 1–2 ml/kg/%BSA.
3 Sodium loss: 200 mmol% BSA m^2.

These estimates may be used as starting points from which to proceed pending laboratory and other data. Calcium, phosphate, magnesium and zinc are important ions and should be included as necessary in any replacement programme either enterally or parenterally.

Nutritional requirements

Within the first few days after the injury protein losses rise and are sustained at high levels, coinciding with a hypermetabolic state which is maximal at about seven days. The aim therefore must be:
1 To reduce hypermetabolism by nursing the patient in a raised ambient temperature of 25–30°C.
2 To provide from an early stage calories and nitrogen sufficient to replenish the high energy expenditure and protein loss; the following amounts are suggested:
   Energy: 20 kcal/kg body wt + 70 kcal/%BSA;
   Protein: 1 g/kg body wt + 3 g/%BSA.

When a nasogastric tube is in place and the intestinal tract is functioning, the major portion of these requirements may be given enterally as a sterile prepared mixture administered by an infusion pump. When the patient feels the desire to eat, this should be encouraged by specially prepared meals attractively presented. In some cases it may be necessary to give some or all of the nutritional requirements intravenously through a long line inserted and maintained with scrupulous sterility. Whichever route or routes is employed, account must be taken of electrolytes, trace elements and vitamin requirements. Sufficient water should be included to prevent the onset of dehydration and a non-ketotic hyperosmolar state. Regular urinary and blood sugar estimations should be performed and, where indicated, a continuous infusion of insulin at an initial rate of 0.02 unit/kg/h should be started and then varied according to biochemical estimations.

Treatment of infection

Measures to control infection include environmental management, aseptic techniques, topical chemotherapy, antibiotics, early surgical excision with grafting, and maintenance of satisfactory nutrition. Because of the problem of diminished host defences and the development of resistant strains of organisms, there is a continuing interest in various forms of immunotherapy.

An additional reason for using plasma as resuscitation fluid may be the resulting enhancement of circulating immune globulin levels during the early stages of care. All antibiotics and chemotherapy must be decided upon in consultation with the microbiologist.

Early surgery

The healing process in a burn wound requires the rejection of necrotic material by the underlying healthy tissue. Natural separation by collagenolysis is a slow process lasting up to six weeks, and during this time invasive infection of the burn wound may increase the depth of tissue necrosis. Early surgical excision and grafting, by replacing dead with living tissue, accelerates wound healing, reduces pain and increases mobility. In addition, successful grafting diminishes toxaemia and hypercatabolism, improves nutrition and enhances the patient's general wellbeing.

Prior consultation between surgeon and anaesthetist helps to decide the timing and extent of the initial procedure. Ideally a start should be considered as soon as fluid resuscitation and correction of anaemia are satisfactory and before serious bacterial proliferation occurs. Assuming that no significant disorder or any major organ system exists, a start may be made on the third to fifth day, possibly limited to 15–20% of the body surface initially.

Excision of a full thickness burn entails complete removal of damaged skin down to vascularized subcutaneous tissue. After haemostasis has been obtained split skin grafts are applied to the raw surface and secured with stitches or clips and dressings. As an alternative some surgeons prefer the tangential excision of successive layers of eschar until domes of fat appear with fine punctate bleeding which demonstrates the presence of living tissue which will sustain a skin graft. The object is to preserve viable dermal tissue, especially in such functionally important areas as the hands.

When adequate graft donor sites are not available mesh grafting is used to extend the healing potential of limited skin resources. Normal split skin grafts are taken and fenestrated by a dermatome to give a mesh of dermal tissue up to three times the area of the original donation. If there is still insufficient skin available and very large areas require temporary cover, porcine skin may be used as a biological dressing. This reduces pain, helps to prepare the excised wound for grafting, and allows time for the healing and regrowth of donor areas. It also reduces the negative nitrogen balance and enables physiotherapy to be started earlier.

ANAESTHESIA IN BURNED PATIENTS

Most patients with major burns require a number of anaesthetics during the various stages of their management. There are several ways of providing safe anaesthesia for burned patients. Sample methods are described here for dealing with two different clinical situations.

Immediate life-saving procedures

The restless, hypoxic patient in pain and distress who requires urgent intubation because of threatened airway obstruction is unsuitable for topical anaesthesia alone. Any form of intravenous induction agent is best avoided until the airway is secured, and an inhalation method is therefore the technique of choice. When combined with topical lignocaine it provides satisfactory intubating conditions under minimal depth of anaesthesia. The local anaesthetic is best applied from a pressurised container, dispensing 10 mg of lignocaine per spray.

Technique

1   Pre-oxygenate the patient with 100% oxygen.
2   Apply ECG electrodes, check BP and insert a free-running infusion. Atropine 0.6 mg is drawn up ready for use.
3   Explain the procedure to the patient and lightly spray the right or left nostril using a total of 30–40 mg lignocaine. Spray the anterior part of the tongue and, in edentulous patients, the maxilla with a further 30 mg lignocaine. Encourage the patient to swallow, thus dispersing the local anaesthetic liquid.
4   If the face is burned apply a gamgee square with an oronasal opening and induce anaesthesia with 50% nitrous oxide/oxygen and increasing concentrations of halothane or enflurane. Insert an airway if required.
5   Interrupt anaesthesia briefly and introduce a laryngoscope to spray sequentially the posterior tongue and vallecula, the cords and the subglottic region, employing 30 mg of lignocaine for each area. The total dose should not exceed 200 mg.
6   Continue anaesthesia for two minutes to allow the local spray to be effective and then introduce a well-lubricated nasal tube; when it is seen in the nasopharynx use Magill forceps to advance it into the trachea. The type of tube is a matter for individual preference.
7   Should the cords be difficult to see, use a fibre-optic bronchoscope inserted through the tube to place the latter in the trachea.

Early excision and grafting

The surgeon and anaesthetist together select the optimum day for the first excision and grafting. When surgery is planned the anaesthetist must have all the clinical and laboratory data made available.

Intragastric feeding should be discontinued for four hours before, and metaclopramide 10 mg given intravenously three hours before induction of anaesthesia. An analgesic premedication should be prescribed unless the patient is already being managed by an opiate infusion. In the presence of tachycardia atropine is avoided but should be available during induction if needed.

The anaesthetist must be sure of the availability of the following:
1   Adequate numbers of experienced staff to help both anaesthetist and surgeon.
2   Two intravenous lines and a sufficient supply of whole blood (three units available in the theatre suite), with filtering, warming and pressurizing facilities. Preferably one intravenous line should be placed centrally for CVP readings.

3 A warm mattress for the operating table and equipment to warm and humidify anaesthetic gases.

4 Monitors for ECG and temperature.

5 A manual or automatic oscillotonometric sphygmomanometer. If the burned area precludes the use of a cuff, intra-arterial monitoring may be possible in a radial or dorsalis pedis vessel.

6 Swab weighing scales or other blood loss measuring device.

The nasogastric tube is aspirated immediately prior to induction and cricoid pressure applied. A suitable intravenous induction–relaxant–analgesic–inhalation sequence may be employed according to the anaesthetist's preference. Suxamethonium must be avoided because of the possible hyperkalaemic response, but atracurium may be used. Intubation may be facilitated by local analgesia to the cords and trachea. It is probably wise to avoid halothane because of the need for repeated anaesthetics.

Blood loss during surgery

Blood loss is greatest during excision of the burned area and the cutting of grafts; a blood transfusion should be running from early in the procedure to replace this loss. It may be necessary to continue the transfusion into the post-operative period because of further loss into the dressings from donor sites. The patient's haemoglobin level should be estimated post-operatively.

Respiratory support

If the patient has a degree of lung damage, a fall in arterial Po_2 after surgery is common, and blood gas checks should be made before and after surgery, with inspired oxygen enrichment provided as required. Rarely, it may be necessary to provide IPPV for a brief period following operation.

Post-operative care

Donor sites are painful and there is a need for adequate analgesia. Metaclopramide may be given six-hourly for 24 hours to improve gastric motility, and feeding can usually be attempted three hours after the end of anaesthesia. During the peri-operative 24-hour period the parenteral calorie intake should be increased to compensate for the reduction of oral or nasogastric intake.

Analgesia for burns dressings

The extent of burn surface area and the patient's pain threshold will influence the amount of analgesia required during wound cleaning, hydrotherapy and dressing.

During the period following admission an intravenous infusion of morphine or papaveretum may have been employed for pain relief, and the amount required will indicate the patient's pain tolerance and the response to opiates. Initial dressings and other painful procedures may be carried out by suitable adjustment of the infusion rate.

Later procedures will need separate periods of fairly deep analgesia. The many techniques which have been devised for this kind of pain relief indicate that none of them is pre-eminently satisfactory. The basic requirements include:

1 Adequate analgesia and patient acceptability.
2 Minimal interference with appetite and food intake.
3 Safety in the absence of a member of the medical staff.
4 Safety when used while the patient is in a saline bath.

A technique which attempts to embody the above criteria includes an intramuscular opiate, with or without metaclopramide, 30 minutes before the procedure. This is followed by the inhalation of non-sleep concentration of 50% nitrous oxide in oxygen (Entonox) during the more painful parts of the treatment. One of the attendants should be detailed to supervise the analgesia, explaining to the patient how to obtain the best use of the inhalation agent. The value of hypnotherapy should not be overlooked and the calm reassuring presence of an experienced nurse goes part of the way towards this in suitable subjects.

Where particular problems exist an anaesthetist should be present to ensure adequate and safe analgesia with intravenous or other techniques, combining sedation and analgesia. Careful notes of the method used are made so that a suitable technique may be re-used on subsequent occasions.

RESPIRATORY DAMAGE

The lung is adversely affected by severe burns even in the absence of inhalation damage. Where the respiratory tract is directly involved by the inhalation of hot, toxic gases the effects are magnified and the subsequent mortality for a given percentage of body surface burn is dramatically increased. It is becoming more evident that, even where there may be little obvious indication of pulmonary involvement, all victims of a conflagration should be considered at risk until proved otherwise.

Although the effects of heat, toxic fumes and explosion may coexist in the same patient it is necessary to look at them separately because of the different problems posed.

Heat

Hot dry gases rapidly lose their heat to the upper airway and may be almost at body temperature on reaching the lower airway. Thus the mucous membranes above the carina are more likely to be damaged than are those below. However, lower airway and lung burns can occur on inhalation of hot steam or from the ignition of an inhaled oxygen–fuel mixture.

Depending on the amount of heat energy transferred, damage to the mucosa will range from erythema and swelling to blistering, desquamation and necrosis with mucosal and submucosal oedema. Within a few hours intraluminal swelling may reach obstructive dimensions. Where burns around the face and neck occur this will compound the internal obstruction by external pressure on the airway. Indeed, even when actual inhalation damage is minimal, oedema of the face, submandibular area and neck may be sufficient to cause obstructive pressure, particularly when aggressive intravenous therapy is in progress.

Smoke

The composition of smoke is complex; it varies according to the materials burned, the amount of oxygen available and the temperature developed in the fire. The effects of inhalation may be considered as general or local, and some patients may be seriously affected in both ways. General systemic effects occur early, but the local respiratory consequences may not arise for some hours or even days after the incident.

General effects

1   Asphyxiation due to the low oxygen and possibly high carbon dioxide content of smoke. Respiratory stimulation from CO_2 may increase the intake of other toxic agents.
2   Systemic toxicity associated with carbon monoxide and cyanide derived from plastic foam.

The most common inhaled toxin is carbon monoxide, generated when inadequate oxygen is available for complete combustion. It has an affinity for haemoglobin 200 times that of oxygen, and an inhaled concentration of 0.1% will convert more than 60% of haemoglobin into carboxyhaemoglobin. There is also a shift to the left of the oxygen dissociation curve, further reducing the amount of oxygen available at cell level, although this effect may be reduced by hypoxic acidosis.

The brain and heart are the organs most affected by the hypoxia and consequent non-respiratory acidosis. An atmosphere of 0.1% CO causes unconsciousness and may be fatal or lead to permanent CNS damage. A detrimental effect on the heart is likely where pre-existing coronary artery disease is present and in these circumstances acute myocardial infarction may ensue.

Respiratory irritants

The following are examples of smoke constituents which may cause tracheobronchial and pulmonary damage:
1   Tars, soot, dust
2   Sulphur dioxide
3   Hydrochloric and hydrocyanic acids
4   Ammonia
5   Aldehydes
6   Nitrogen dioxide
7   Toluene diisocyanate

When such irritants are inhaled in significant quantities there may be a sequence of immediate coughing, laryngospasm and salivation giving way to desiccation of the oropharyngeal mucosa, increasing hoarseness and bronchospasm.

The effects on the lung parenchyma usually take some time to develop. In some cases these may be relatively mild with a moderate degree of hypoxaemia lasting a few days, while in others there may be the full picture of acute respiratory distress needing maximal support. Between these extremes there is found a considerable range of clinical pathology.

Postmortem studies of smoke damaged patients who do not survive demonstrate a range of injuries. In the air passages oedema, submucosal haemorrhages and bronchorrhoea are seen with the naked eye, while the lungs are heavy and congested with blood and fluid oozing from the sectioned surface.

When the damage has been severe, the effects on respiratory function are threefold:

1   There is an increased resistance to airflow within the entire lower respiratory tract due to bronchospasm, oedema and intraluminal fluid.

2   Patchy alveolar collapse and pulmonary oedema result in disturbed ventilation–perfusion ratios and a reduced diffusing capacity for oxygen.

3   Effective compliance falls, due to reduction of alveolar volume. Those alveoli which are being ventilated have an increased surface tension from deficient or altered surfactant and thus require a higher opening pressure.

As a result of increased airflow resistance and diminished compliance there is a marked increase in the work of breathing. Before the full onset of these effects, in the early post-burn period, tachypnoeic hyperventilation may be seen with a reduction in $Pa\text{CO}_2$, but this is followed by alveolar hypoventilation. There is usually an early and continued downward progression of the $Pa\text{O}_2$.

Infection is a common complication; therapeutic measures such as tracheal intubation or tracheostomy increase the likelihood of bacterial invasion.

Explosion

The degree of lung damage which results from an explosion depends on the amplitude and spread of the induced pressure change. Thus the deflagration and detonation of a fuel/air mixture may produce a wave profile which is less destructive than that of a high explosive device, although the effects are similar qualitatively. The degree of injury will also be affected by the location of the victim relative to the epicentre and by the possible shielding effect of intervening structures and furniture.

When there is full exposure to a steep over-pressure waveform, this will result in the generation of high pressure differentials in the lungs. Diffuse pulmonary haemorrhage, alveolar wall rupture, pneumothorax, pneumomediastinum and air embolism are the common sequelae, and these injuries carry a high mortality. Major blood vessels and bronchi may be damaged, and the extent of intrathoracic bleeding is often lethal. Intra-abdominal structures, particularly the large bowel, are frequently injured at the same time; subserosal haemorrhage, linear tears and full thickness perforations are very common. Solid structures (liver, spleen) are rarely involved in blast injuries although they are sometimes damaged by flying or falling objects.

The possibility of occult injury must always be considered when the victims of explosion are seen.

Diagnosis of inhalation damage

Respiratory distress may become apparent very quickly or the problem may manifest itself only after an extended time. If there are signs of serious involvement of the upper airway the patient must be intubated before oedema makes this manoeuvre difficult and dangerous. Other diagnostic and therapeutic measures take second place.

History and examination

The history of the incident, type and location of the fire, amount of visible smoke, duration of involvement and the proximity of the face to burning material all provide useful information. Other features to be looked for during the first 24 hours include:
1   Burns of face and neck with singeing of nasal hairs
2   Soot particles in nose, mouth and sputum
3   Desiccation or blistering of tongue, mouth and pharynx
4   Cyanosis, restlessness and confusion
5   Hoarseness possibly leading to aphonia
6   Inspiratory stridor (upper airway) or expiratory grunting (lung)
7   Retrosternal pain or tightness
8   Auscultation: lungs—bronchospasm; larynx—increasingly harsh breath sounds

Investigations

Blood gases

The effects of burn injury upon the blood gases were referred to above. Blood gas analysis and the Aa gradient should be recorded frequently.

Carboxyhaemoglobin

The so-called 'cherry red' appearance is an inconsistent sign and carboxyhaemoglobin should always be looked for in the first specimen of blood from a patient who has been involved in a fire, especially in an enclosed space. Significantly toxic levels may be found, requiring immediate treatment. Less toxic amounts could indicate:
1   the possibility of previously higher levels causing cerebral hypoxia and brain damage;
2   the concomitant inhalation of lung irritants, thus requiring continued observation of lung function.

Late estimation is a less reliable index, especially if the patient has been treated with a high oxygen concentration, since the latter displaces carbon monoxide from the haemoglobin molecule.

Chest radiology

Severe damage may cause early radiological changes, but a normal chest x-ray on admission does not preclude lung damage. It is more common for a delay of 12–24 hours to occur before diffuse alveolar shadowing displays the effects of smoke inhalation or blast injuries.

Fibre-optic bronchoscopy

This examination, carried out under local anaesthesia with a 5 mm bronchoscope, can be of particular value. It may reveal tracheal and bronchial damage from heat or irritant fumes in patients where such effects might not otherwise have been diagnosed.

The use of the fibre-optic bronchoscope to facilitate endotracheal intubation is referred to on page 48.

Lung scan

The injection of a saline solution of xenon^{-133} into an arm vein is normally followed by a lung excretion phase lasting up to 90–150 sec, as shown by serial gamma camera scans; prolongation of this wash-out phase may indicate the presence of acute lung damage.

Management of respiratory damage

Fire or blast victims with obvious respiratory problems need urgent airway care and possibly ventilatory support on admission. Similarly, unconscious patients having suspected carbon monoxide or other systemic poisoning require intubation and ventilation with an oxygen-rich mixture. These patients risk further brain damage by the onset of post-hypoxic fits; the administration of thiopentone or phenytoin should be considered after ventilatory and fluid therapy have been initiated.

Most patients with blast or inhalation damage develop respiratory difficulties only after resuscitation has been under way for some time. Typically, patients who have been involved in explosions do not demonstrate signs of respiration inadequacy for 24–48 hours. They must all be observed closely during this initial period for increased airflow resistance or evidence of parenchymal damage which, either singly or in combination, may be sufficient to warrant intervention.

The details of treatment are as described in the section on ARDS. Endotracheal intubation or tracheostomy, humidification, IPPV with oxygen enrichment and PEEP may all be required. In addition bronchodilators and antibiotics may be required, and methylprednisolone (30 mg/kg 6-hourly) has been recommended, but without conclusive benefit. If they are used not more than three doses should be given.

BURNS IN CHILDREN

In children, although the overall pathophysiology and management remain broadly similar to that of adults, there are particular points to be taken into consideration.

1   Appropriate charts and tables will be needed to determine surface areas, physiological normals, fluid and calorie requirements according to age and weight. These are available in textbooks specifically devoted to paediatrics and to burns management.

2   Intravenous resuscitation is required if there is more than 10% BSA, as against 15% in the adult.

3   For intravenous therapy a cut-down will usually be needed.

4   The infant kidney excretes a more dilute urine from the relatively large extravascular space. There is less ability to conserve water and rapid dehydration may ensue.

5   The child has a larger surface area relative to weight, and thus may be expected to lose more heat and water to its surroundings.

6   The smaller diameter airways make obstruction a greater threat in the event of inhalation damage. Endotracheal tubes are easily kinked or dislodged, and tracheostomy is more likely to cause sequelae.

7   Children seem to be more prone to certain complications:
cerebral oedema with convulsions
hypothermia
hypoglycaemia
metabolic acidosis
hypertension

8   In children under two years excision and grafting are less often carried out except for some important areas, thus repeated dressings and saline baths are needed, with special attention to analgesia requirements. For this purpose ketamine is a useful agent given intravenously or intramuscularly.

9   The particular psychological needs of children must be catered for.

10   Children require proportionally greater energy and protein intake than adults. This is calculated from the formula:
Energy: 60 kcal/kg body wt + 35 kcal/%BSA;
Protein: 3 g/kg body wt + 1 g/%BSA.

SOME EARLY COMPLICATIONS OF BURNS

Oliguria and renal failure

Following the occurrence of serious burn injury there is a multiple assault on the kidney, including hypovolaemia, hypotension, vasospasm, haemoconcentration, raised antidiuretic hormone secretion and free plasma haemoglobin. Rapid and adequate fluid replacement is usually sufficient to preserve reasonable function and prevent major damage. However, such factors as a delay in resuscitation, excessive haemolysis or muscle involvement may tip the balance towards acute renal failure.

In the burned patient renal failure creates particular problems with fluid balance. The patient will continue to lose a large and unpredictable amount of fluid from the burned tissue, and this must be replaced. The problems created by haemoglobinuria and myoglobinuria have been referred to earlier. Generous allowance must be made for insensible losses and mannitol 0.5 mg/kg may be given to aid diuresis. Where possible the patient should be nursed on a weighing bed although this will not demonstrate fluid shifts, which may present as oedema. Frequent haematocrit measurements are essential and central venous pressure monitoring may be helpful, where practicable. In other respects the diagnosis and management of renal failure is as described on page 17.

Gastroduodenal erosion and ulceration

Varying degrees of erosive gastritis or duodenitis are common in severe injury. These may progress to frank ulceration, a condition classically described by Curling in 1842, although others before him had noted the occurrence of gastrointestinal ulceration. Many aetiologies have been suggested, and although the role of gastric acid secretion appears dominant, such ulceration may occur in segments of bowel not directly influenced by gastric acidity, especially when there is an elevated blood urea. If it is not prevented and vigorously treated, haematemesis or perforation may occur.

Neutralization of gastric acid secretion with two-hourly antacid orally or through nasogastric tube has considerably reduced the incidence of stress erosion. The use of H_2 blocking agents such as cimetidine and ranitidine has further helped. This preventative therapy is continued until enteral feeding has been well established.

Bronchopneumonia

Bronchopneumonia may occur in three broad categories of burn injury:
1 Patients with known inhalation damage who develop one of a wide range of effects from the fairly mild to the severe and fatal.
2 Patients without a definitive history of inhalation but in whom progressive pulmonary insufficiency is followed by the onset of infection.
3 Patients in whom there has been no possibility of inhalation damage but who develop a late onset of bronchopneumonia. This is more likely in the elderly and debilitated or those with previous bronchopulmonary disease.

Apart from the possible effects of blast or smoke inhalation, other factors have a role in the development of pulmonary infection. It has been shown in experimental animals that burn wound sepsis reduces the clearance of bacteria from the tracheobronchial tree. Haematogenous bacterial spread may also play a part since the organisms cultured from sputum are similar to those found in the burn wound in about 30% of cases. In addition there is lowered host resistance because of reduced serum immunoglobulin levels, altered neutrophil function and nutritional deficiency. As previously described, patients with trunk burns may have a decreased vital capacity and this will set the scene for sputum retention, atelectasis and bronchopneumonia, especially in the older age group. Finally, interference with normal barriers to infection by intubation or tracheostomy may also be a potent cause of bacterial lung invasion.

Treatment

When infection occurs, treatment should include the antibiotics which are recommended by the clinical microbiologist; humidified oxygen and physiotherapy are always required, and the use of bronchodilators may be suggested by the physical signs. If the blood gases are not improved by these measures, intubation, tracheobronchial toilet and possibly controlled ventilation should be considered. However, in the elderly patient with a large BSA such intensive therapy may be inappropriate.

Septicaemia

Episodes of bacteraemia occur in a majority of patients with over 30% burns. In some cases bacteria enter the blood as early as five hours after the burn, possibly gaining access from hypoxic bowel rather than from the burn site. Bacteraemia may progress to the full picture of septicaemia with positive blood culture, raised core temperature, reduced cardiac output, oliguria and hypoxia.

Treatment should be started with appropriate antibiotic therapy and the usual support provided for cardiovascular, lung and renal function.

Disseminated intravascular coagulation

Platelets and coagulation factors decrease early in thermal injury, and this may indicate a raised consumption through disseminated intravascular coagulation (DIC). The onset of infection may convert a mild or latent DIC into a more florid coagulopathy. Management is described on page 94.

CARE OF PATIENTS UNLIKELY TO RECOVER

There is a group of patients with major severe burns and possibly inhalation damage who have little chance of survival. Vigorous treatment may therefore be inappropriate on humanitarian grounds, and a decision concerning this should be made by senior members of the burns team.

The emphasis must then be towards analgesia and comfort for the patient together with support and explanation for the relatives. Sips of water or small cubes of ice may be given orally, and simple intravenous infusion of 5% dextrose will also help reduce thirst and provide a line for analgesia. Without aggressive resuscitation those patients with upper airway damage may not survive to develop signs of obstruction. However, when this is a threat the patient should be nasally intubated so as to reduce the distress which would be caused by untreated asphyxia. One or two close relatives may be allowed to sit with the patient if they so wish and adequate spiritual support offered should this be desired.

ELECTRICAL BURNS

The severity of these burns depends on the amount of electrical energy passing through the body, which in turn is related to the applied voltage, the resistance in the circuit and the duration of current flow. The resulting burns assume clinical significance where the patient has not been killed outright by the cardiorespiratory effects at the time of the incident. Although most of the damage arises from the heat generated by the current, some of the adverse effects are believed to be related to the electrical current itself.

Characteristically, the burns are severe and deep with muscle damage, myoglobinaemia and impairment of renal function. Unless there has been sparking and arc formation, as associated with high voltage supply, there may be minimal external signs of the amount of destruction of deeper tissues. On the other hand, burns arising from the brief radiant heat of a flash-over in a high tension circuit may not be deep because usually the current does not pass through the body. However, the victim may be spattered with fused metal or be involved in a secondary fire.

Although the BSA may be less significant, the treatment of electrical burns follows the same pattern as ordinary thermal burns. In the immediate phase renal function requires special care because of the muscle damage; the risk of swelling within myofascial compartments may call for early fasciotomy.

CHEMICAL BURNS

Chemical burns tend to arise mainly in industry where the use of corrosive substances is a part of numerous production processes. Although termed 'burns' the damage is induced chemically rather than thermally. However, in the cases of metallic sodium and potassium, which burst into flame on contact with water, and phosphorus which ignites in air at room temperature, thermal skin damage may occur.

A major problem with some chemicals is absorption from the skin to cause systemic poisoning. A number of such substances is listed in Table 5 along with the organs or systems likely to be adversely affected.

Table 5. Chemicals absorbed from the skin

Chemical	Adverse effects
Phenols, cresols	CNS, liver, kidney
Lysol	Red cells
Hydrofluoric acid	Reduced serum calcium and magnesium
Formic acid	Kidney
Chromic acid	Kidney
All acids and alkalis	Acidosis or alkalosis
Methyl bromide	CNS

Local treatment

There are 25 to 30 fairly common agents which may cause skin burns on contact, each with its characteristic type of damage. Different groups may require specific neutralizing agents and immediate local treatment. In general terms, copious lavage with water is a useful first measure, except in the case of sodium and potassium which must be covered with oil.

General treatment

The area of damaged skin should be reckoned by the use of body charts, and appropriate fluid resuscitation begun together with other measures as described under thermal burns. Depending on the chemical substance, absorption may require to be monitored and treated accordingly. In the case of some acids or ammonia, inhalation of the vapour can cause tracheobronchial and lung damage. Chest radiographs and serial blood gas estimation are needed during the first 48 hours.

References

Artz, C.P., Moncrief, J.A. & Pruitt, B.A. (1979) *Burns—A Team Approach.* 583 pp. Philadelphia: W.B. Saunders Co.

Carson, J.S. (1979) *Treatment of Burns.* 339 pp. London: Chapman and Hall.

Davies, J.W.L. (1982) *Physiological Responses to Burning Injury.* 649 pp. London: Academic Press.

Heidman, M. (1979) The effect of thermal injury on haemodynamic, respiratory and haematological variables in relation to complement activation. *Journal of Trauma,* **19,** 239–243.

Hilton, J.G. (1981) Effect of fluid resuscitation on total fluid loss following thermal injury. *Surgery, Gynecology and Obstetrics,* **152,** 441–447.

Humble, R.P. (1982) *Clinical Burn Therapy.* 567 pp. Boston: John Wright, PSG Inc.

Jenkinson, L.R. (1982) Fluid replacement in burns. A burns calculator. *Annals of the Royal College of Surgeons,* **64,** 336–338.

McCaughey, W., Coppel, D. & Dundee, J.W. (1973) Blast injuries to the lungs. *Anaesthesia,* **28,** 2–9.

Zawacki, B.E., Azen, S.P., Imbus, S.H. & Chang, Y.T.L. (1979) Multifactorial probit analysis of mortality in burned patients. *Annals of Surgery,* **189,** 1–5.

8

Coma and Disorders of Consciousness after Trauma

N.E.F. CARTLIDGE

In practice patients with disorders of consciousness after trauma present some of the most difficult problems in management. The emotional impact of the accidental injury, the panic aroused by the sight of an unconscious and perhaps bloody casualty, and the rush to obtain help all may blur the description of what actually happened to the patient between injury and admission to hospital. Transfer to a specialist unit further compounds the problem and the end result is that details of the accident, the patient's consciousness level after injury and the evolution of subsequent events is often lacking. The need for a complete early examination, attention to the patient's airway, treatment of shock, and assessment of the level of consciousness cannot be overemphasized.

This chapter will concern itself primarily with the causes and the early assessment of patients with disordered consciousness after trauma. The problems of delayed deterioration in consciousness, prolonged coma, investigations and brain death will also be considered.

Pathophysiology of disordered consciousness

A detailed description of the pathophysiology of consciousness and coma is beyond the scope of this chapter, and only a few brief comments will be included. Normal consciousness requires an interaction between the reticular activating system of the brain stem and the cerebral cortex. The reticular activating system is responsible for arousal or alertness and the cerebral cortex for the content of consciousness or the awareness of self and environment. Impairment of consciousness can result from lesions affecting the reticular formation, the reticular formation–cortical connections or the cerebral cortex. Coma resulting from a head injury probably results from a disordered reticular formation, and drugs produce coma by their effect on the reticular formation. Hypoxia and hypotension may produce coma by diffuse depression of the cerebral cortex. A unilateral supratentorial lesion such as a subdural or extradural haematoma will only produce coma when there is diencephalic or brain stem damage resulting from herniation of structures through the tentorial hiatus. As will be seen later, it should be possible on the basis of the pattern of physical signs to determine whether the disordered consciousness in an individual case has resulted from reticular formation or brain stem damage, diffuse cortical depression, or rostro-caudal herniation from a supratentorial lesion.

CAUSES OF DISORDERED CONSCIOUSNESS

Following injury there is often a natural tendency to assume that impairment of consciousness has resulted from head injury. This is only one of the many factors which may be operative, and some of these are listed in Table 6. In the early assessment of the patient after trauma only the first three of these factors need to be taken into account, and the first priority is to determine which of these is the main contributing factor. Haldane's now famous statement that 'anoxia not only stops the machine but wrecks the machinery' was made in an article in the British Medical Journal in 1919 and is as pertinent today as it was then. The first priority is basic First Aid and the maintenance of respiration and circulation. The importance of hypoxia and the dangers of the 'second accident' cannot be emphasized too often. Deteriorating consciousness after trauma is more likely to be due to hypoxia than to an acute intracranial haematoma.

In general, it is safer to assume that any disorder of respiration or circulation which is present is more likely to be the *cause* of disordered consciousness rather than the result of associated brain injury. Neurogenic disorders of respiration are exceptional in patients who have not suffered severe brain injury and neurogenic vasomotor abnormalities are usually only seen as an agonal phenomenon. Massive pituitary damage secondary to brain injury could theoretically produce 'neurogenic hypotension' but clinical examples of this are extreme rarities. A good working rule is that shock means a major injury elsewhere than to the head.

Effects of coincidental treatment

Another early priority is to attempt to determine any therapy that the patient may have been given. This applies not only to drugs given after admission to

Table 6. Factors affecting consciousness in the patient after trauma

1. Head trauma:
   (a) Primary impact damage
   (b) Complicating cerebral oedema
   (c) Intracranial haematoma

2. Hypoxia

3. Hypotension

4. Drugs:
   Analgesics, sedatives

5. Metabolic disorders:
   Renal failure, hepatic failure

6. Miscellaneous:
   e.g. fat embolism, DIC, etc

hospital but also to previous therapy which may have been given at the site of trauma or in the ambulance. Such therapy may be necessary in the patient who has multiple injuries, and if at all possible attempts should be made to assess the patient's conscious level *before* any drugs are given. A detailed neurological assessment is relatively easy to perform with experience, and once basic First Aid has been given, and if no life-threatening conditions require urgent treatment, then this should be performed.

THE ASSESSMENT OF THE UNCONSCIOUS PATIENT

History

In many instances one is faced with a traumatized patient for whom no history is available, and there should be *no delay* in moving on to the examination and the neurological assessment. At the same time attempts should be made to obtain history from relatives, witnesses or the ambulance men who brought the patient to hospital. The events which occurred at the time of the accident may not be particularly helpful, though it should be remembered that occasionally accidents may be *caused* by an event such as a spontaneous subarachnoid haemorrhage which in itself may be affecting the patient's level of consciousness. Of considerable importance is the state of the patient's conscious level when he was first seen after the injury, and such questions as 'Did the patient ever talk, open his eyes, or move?' should be asked of all people who have had prior contact with the patient. If the patient has suffered a seizure this may be relevant and particular note made of whether this was generalized or focal. It cannot be stressed too strongly that any information concerning the evolution of the patient's state is of considerable importance.

General assessment

The general assessment may be of particular value in indicating the presence or absence of a head injury and may even be helpful in determining the severity of brain injury. However, severe brain injuries may occur in the absence of any obvious external signs. The location of an acute intracranial haematoma can be more confidently related to the point of external impact than to localizing neurological signs, and hence recording of the external signs of injury is an important part of the baseline assessment. The site of bruises and the position of lacerations on the skull should particularly be noted. Lacerations which overlie a skull fracture indicate a compound injury which requires antibiotic prophylaxis. Ecchymotic discolouration of the skin over the mastoid process (Battle's sign) may suggest the presence of a fracture of the petrous temporal bone and this, together with bleeding from the external auditory meatus on that side, strongly suggests compound fracture of the floor of the middle fossa. Bleeding from the nose suggests the possibility of a fracture through the anterior cranial fossa and careful observation should be made to see if this is accompanied by a cerebrospinal fluid leak. A subconjunctival haemorrhage stopping at the sclerocorneal junction accompanied by bleeding from the nose is a further pointer to a possible compound fracture of the anterior cranial fossa. A bruise near the outer edge of the eyebrow with a dilated pupil on that side suggests that the pupillary dilatation may be due to an optic nerve injury.

Retinoscopy

Examination of the optic fundi should be made, if only to have a baseline assessment against which later examination can be compared. Retinal haemorrhages are not uncommon after head injury and are of no particular significance. Papilloedema is excessively uncommon in the early stages following head injury, though its later development may be a useful sign of raised intracranial pressure arising from cerebral oedema or an expanding intracranial haematoma.

Meningism

The neck should be examined to determine if it is supple, and in the early stages after a head injury the presence of neck stiffness usually indicates a traumatic subarachnoid haemorrhage. If there is no associated Kernig's sign the neck rigidity may be due to tonsilar herniation through the foramen magnum. In deep coma neck stiffness may be absent despite the presence of blood in the subarachnoid space.

The development of neck stiffness when this was previously absent is a particularly important sign, suggesting either the development of meningitis or an intracranial haematoma.

Table 7a. The neurological assessment of the patient in coma

1. General assessment:
   Skull
   Ears
   Fundi
   Signs of meningism

2. Level of consciousness:
   The Glasgow coma scale
   (a) Verbal responses
   (b) Eye opening
   (c) Motor responses

3. Brainstem function:
   (a) Pupillary reactions
   (b) Spontaneous eye movements
   (c) Oculocephalic responses
   (d) Oculovestibular responses
   (e) Corneal responses
   (f) Respiratory pattern

4. Motor function:
   (a) Deep tendon reflexes
   (b) Skeletal muscle tone

Level of consciousness

Until relatively recently there has been no satisfactory and generally accepted method for assessing level of consciousness. The so-called 'Glasgow Coma Scale' has now become widely accepted and provides a relatively easy method

Table 7b. Glasgow coma scale

INSTITUTE OF NEUROLOGICAL SCIENCES, GLASGOW OBSERVATION CHART					
NAME				**DATE**	
				TIME	
RECORD No.					

C O M A	Eyes open	Spontaneously		Eyes closed by swelling = C
		To speech		
		To pain		
		None		
	Best verbal response	Orientated		Endotracheal tube or tracheostomy = T
		Confused		
		Inappropriate Words		
		Incomprehensible Sounds		
S C A L E		None		
	Best motor response	Obey commands		Usually record the best arm response
		Localise pain		
		Flexion to pain		
		Extension to pain		
		None		

Pupil scale (m.m.):
1
2
3
4
5
6
7
8

Blood pressure and Pulse rate: 240 230 220 210 200 190 180 170 160 150 140 130 120 110 100 90 80 70 60 50 40 30 20

Respiration: 10

Temperature °C: 40 39 38 37 36 35 34 33 32 31 30

PUPILS	right	Size		+ reacts
		Reaction		— no reaction
	left	Size		c. eye closed
		Reaction		

LIMB MOVEMENT	ARMS	Normal power		Record right (R) and left (L) separately if there is a difference between the two sides.
		Mild weakness		
		Severe weakness		
		Spastic flexion		
		Extension		
		No response		
	LEGS	Normal power		
		Mild weakness		
		Severe weakness		
		Extension		
		No response		

of assessing conscious level (Table 7). It is based on three responses: those of eye opening, motor response and verbal response. As the term 'response' implies, the patient is given a stimulus, either verbal or painful, and the relevant reaction noted. The traditional painful stimulus of sternal pressure or pinching the skin should be avoided for the simple reason that they may bruise the patient. Supraorbital pressure or nail bed pressure with a pen or coin have the advantage that they are very painful, easy to perform and do not mark the skin.

The importance of the scale is that it is easy to perform, has a high inter-observer reliability and is hierarchical, i.e., the lower the score, the greater the depth of coma. The ease by which the scale may be scored enables serial observation to be made, and this is of considerable importance in assessing change in conscious level.

Most hospital records have now included in their charts a simplified version of the scale to allow serial scoring in the patient with impairment of consciousness.

Brain stem function

In an acute situation it may not be possible to perform a detailed examination of the brain stem reflexes. However, these are an important part of the routine assessment of the unconscious patient and disturbance of the brain stem reflexes may occur in a variety of different clinical situations. In the patient with rostro-caudal herniation from a supratentorial haematoma, there is typically a unilateral third nerve palsy with dilatation of the pupil. Any drug given in sufficient quantity to affect conscious level will paralyse those brain stem reflexes concerned with eye movement. Finally, the criteria for brain death include as a prerequisite absence of the brain stem reflexes. For these reasons the individual brain stem reflexes will be described and the techniques for their examination detailed.

Pupils

The pupils should be examined for size, equality and reaction to light. Before concluding that the pupillary light reflex is absent, a bright light should be used and the movement of the iris assessed with a hand-lens. Unilateral absence of the pupillary light reflex may result from an optic nerve lesion and this may be differentiated from the midriasis of a third nerve palsy by the differences between consensual and direct reflex. Disorders of consciousness resulting from drugs rarely affect the pupils. Spurious changes in the size of the pupils or the pupillary reactions may be observed in patients with iris disease, those who have received midriatic or cycloplegic agents, or pre-existing disorders such as the Adie syndrome. Muscle relaxants have no effect upon pupillary reactions to light or accommodation.

Spontaneous eye movements

The assessment of spontaneous or reflex eye movements is one of the most valuable components of the examination of brain stem function, and full knowledge of the anatomical pathways subserving eye movements is necessary in order to interpret the variety of abnormalities. In the unconscious patient, the spontaneous rapid eye movements of the awake individual are absent. In light coma, there will often be slow conjugate or dysconjugate roving eye movements either horizontally or vertically. Full spontaneous movements require participation of the entire conjugate gaze systems of the brain stem and a full horizontal excursion of both eyes indicates that the pons and the mid-brain are relatively intact. In deep coma from any cause, including drug overdose coma, the eyes are fixed; muscle relaxants have the same effect. In the assessment of the comatose patient, the effects of *all* drugs must be considered since they are a frequent cause of misunderstanding.

A slight divergence of the eyes is not uncommon at all levels of obtundation. Conjugate deviation of the eyes to one side may be indicative of either a hemisphere or brain stem lesion, and when persistent indicates a paralysis of gaze.

Oculocephalic response

In the absence of spontaneous eye movements it is important to try to get some assessment of reflex eye movement. The oculocephalic response or 'dolls head' manoeuvre is the simplest test of reflex eye movement but may be absent without brain stem damage and often requires keen observation. Another disadvantage is that the test may be difficult to perform in a patient who is intubated. Normally when the head is rotated horizontally to one side, under the influence of the labyrinths the eyes deviate briskly and conjugately to the opposite side. Full horizontal conjugate excursion on head rotation indicates normal functioning of the labyrinths, eighth nerves, conjugate lateral gaze centres, medial longitudinal fasciculi, oculomotor nerves and ocular muscles and rules out *a gross lesion of the brain stem* as a cause of coma. The responses are characteristically depressed in coma due to drugs and brisk in diffuse hemisphere lesions producing coma.

Oculovestibular response

Though more time-consuming to perform, the oculovestibular response gives a more accurate assessment of reflex eye movements as the movements are usually easy to visualize. It is mandatory to examine the external auditory meatus to ensure it is not blocked with wax or blood-clot before performing the test, and the best responses are obtained with ice-cold water. Although as little as 5–10 ml may produce a response, as much as 100 ml should be used before deciding a response is absent. Four grades of response may be recognized:
1 Nystagmus
2 Tonic deviation
3 Impaired deviation
4 No response

In a normal alert individual nystagmus will be seen. The quick phase of the nystagmus requires cortex/brain stem connections; in coma due to a diffuse cortical process, the quick phase of the nystagmus is absent and the slow phase predominates with the result that the eyes are forcibly drawn to the stimulated side (so-called tonic deviation). Symmetrical tonic deviation indicates preservation of brain stem function and is characteristic of diffuse hemisphere lesions producing coma. Asymmetrical deviation is characteristic of a focal brain stem lesion, though it may be seen in patients who have taken or been given any of a variety of sedative drugs. Absent oculovestibular responses bilaterally indicate either a profound brain stem disturbance, drugs (including muscle relaxants), or bilateral middle ear pathology.

Corneal responses

The corneal reflexes are usually preserved other than in deep coma. Exaggerated corneal responses with grimacing are characteristic of patients in the vegetative state (see below). Asymmetry of the corneal responses may be of value in localization.

Respiratory pattern

A variety of abnormalities of respiration may be seen in coma. The best recognized abnormality is that of Cheyne–Stokes respiration which, contrary to common belief, usually indicates that the patient is not in imminent danger of death. It should be emphasized that breathing which is stertorous has no special neurological significance and is due to partial respiratory obstruction.

Motor function

As discussed above in the section dealing with the Glasgow coma scale, abnormalities of function are of hierarchical value. That is to say, no motor response is 'worse' than an extensor motor response. In man, the pathological lesions producing decerebrate (extensor) or decorticate (flexor) responses do not follow such precise anatomical correlates as in Sherringtonian experiments and extensor responses may be seen in cortical, subcortical or brain stem lesions. The terms decerebrate or decorticate should not be applied to man.

Motor response and posture

The motor response is of particular importance in the neurological assessment of the unconscious patient because of the *localizing value of asymmetry*. Asymmetry of motor function in coma almost invariably suggests focal pathology, and the development of asymmetry of motor responses is a particularly important sign.

The posture of the limbs may give a clue to asymmetry, but this often simply reflects the position in which the patient is lying. A painful stimulus should be applied to right and left limbs separately to compare the responses, and the movement of right and left limbs to supraorbital pressure should be assessed. Asymmetry of facial grimacing may be a useful localizing sign.

The tendon reflexes are of limited value in the assessment of motor function. They may be present even in patients who otherwise fulfil the criteria of brain death, and in unconscious patients it is often difficult to detect asymmetry. The planter response retains its localizing value.

Muscle tone may be scored hierarchically through normal, flexor, extensor to flaccid. Flaccid muscle tone may be seen not only in severe brain damage but also in patients who have received drugs. Asymmetry of motor tone should be sought not only in the limbs but also in the eyelids. Spontaneous motor activity such as myoclonus, seizures or other involuntary movements may be of diagnostic value. Focal seizures have the same implication as focal signs.

Spinal injuries in an unconscious patient may manifest themselves by a discrepancy between motor responses and eye opening or verbal responses. A patient who eye-opens and groans to pain yet remains flaccid with no motor responses is likely to have a cervical cord injury. Similarly, movement of the arms but not of the legs to pain suggests lower cord damage.

The above scheme for the neurological assessment of the unconscious patient should, with practice, take a relatively short period of time. At the very least regular serial assessments of conscious level using the Glasgow coma scale should be made and, where at all possible, a full neurological assessment performed at least once daily.

INVESTIGATION OF HEAD INJURY

Skull x-rays

Theoretically, skull x-rays taken at an early stage in the management of a head injury should be of value in anticipating complications, and ideally they should be obtained as soon as possible after resuscitation and initial assessment. In practice, this is often more difficult. Often the patient with trauma is admitted at night when hospital staffing is at a low ebb and where a radiographer has to be called from home. If the patient is restless and confused the radiographs may be of little value and often these will have to be repeated at a later stage when he is more cooperative. For these reasons it may not be possible to obtain skull x-rays on all patients after trauma.

The presence of a skull fracture does not relate to the severity of brain injury. Skull fractures indicate the presence of damage to the skull but not necessarily the brain. However, they are present in three-quarters of all patients who develop an extradural haematoma which indicates the need for careful observation of all patients with a skull fracture. The position in children is a little different, as the presence of a skull fracture alone, without clinical evidence of damage to the central nervous system, is of little significance.

Echoencephalography

Echoencephalography is a safe bedside technique and at first glance a very attractive screening test for intracranial pathology. However, a midline echo can be obtained only after very considerable practice, and without this the investigation may be misleading. The error may be as high as 10% in recognizing displacement of midline structures, and this makes the investigations scarcely adequate for the discrimination required of it.

Nevertheless, echoencephalography does have a useful though limited role; for example, when a patient with multiple injuries needs sedation, such as in the case of controlled ventilation for a major chest injury. Ordinary observation may not be feasible, and serial echograms may help to demonstrate the development of intracranial haematoma.

Specific neuroradiological investigations

For many years cerebral angiography was the definitive diagnostic procedure in the management of patients with suspected head injuries. It has now been superseded by computerized axial tomography—the CT scan. In addition to being non-invasive, the scan gives more information about precise pathology and it can differentiate between haematoma, oedema and infarction which the angiogram is unable to do. But in spite of the considerable diagnostic benefits of the scan, its overall contribution in the management of head injuries must inevitably be limited because of the logistical problems in their management. Thus, of the deaths that occur from head injury in the United Kingdom, 40% occur before the patients reach hospital and 20% of the total die in hospital before they can be admitted. Furthermore, not all centres which admit patients with multiple trauma have a CT scan available, and the expense of siting a CT scan in every district general hospital which admits patients after trauma would be enormous.

The CT scan can create problems of its own. It may reveal lesions that were not suspected clinically and these may pose problems in management. With increasing frequency temporal lobe contusion has been diagnosed and this raises the difficult decision as to whether or not excision should be carried out. In fact, surgery is seldom required and the decision should be made on clinical rather than radiological grounds. Numerous studies, however, have confirmed the theoretical expectation that computerized tomography reduces the morbidity from invasive investigations and from exploratory surgery, without influencing overall mortality.

Indications for CT scanning

The most obvious indication for computerized tomography is a progressive deterioration in the neurological state that is not dramatic enough to threaten life immediately. Another circumstance in which such investigation is important is where the history is uncertain and the patient remains unconscious for no obvious reason. Likewise, scanning is useful in patients whose management, for one reason or another, involves techniques that interfere with the normal assessment procedures. It is important to emphasize the caveat that one normal investigation is no guarantee against later complication, and serial scanning may sometimes be called for. In CT scanning fresh blood is seen as a dense white image which is biconvex if extradural (Figure 18). Oedema is less dense than normal brain whilst contusions have a mottled appearance. The density of a clot generally

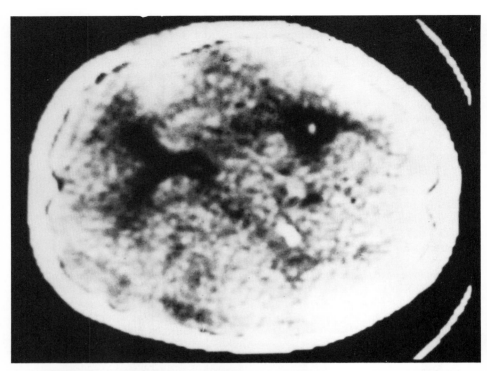

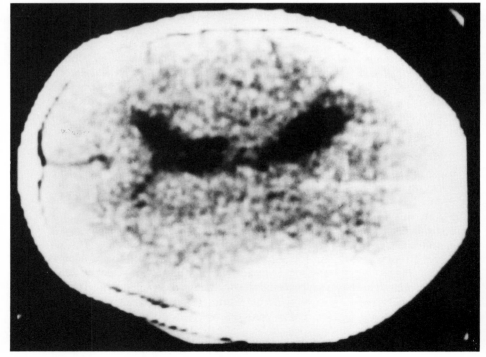

Figure 18. Left-sided extradural haematoma with shift of the ventricular system.   Figure 19. Isodense haematoma with displacement of the midline structures.

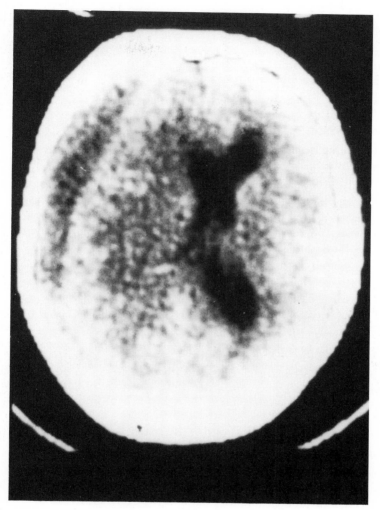

Figure 20. Chronic subdural haematoma with midline shift of the ventricular system.

decreases with age and may sometimes be isodense with adjacent brain; such a clot may not be recognized other than as a displacement of the midline structures (Figure 19) and may be missed altogether if bilateral haematomas prevent any such displacement. A chronic subdural haematoma is less dense than brain and, if wholly fluid, its outline is biconvex (Figure 20).

Angiography may still be indicated when scans are equivocal, or in suspected vascular lesions such as traumatic carotid thrombosis or cortico-cavernous fistula.

Other investigations

Ventriculography

This involves the introduction of a positive or negative contrast medium into the lateral ventricles through a burr hole prior to radiological examination. The technique is rarely performed nowadays as it has been superseded by the CT scan.

Lumbar puncture

This technique has no place in the diagnosis or management of most head injuries. Indeed, if it is carried out indiscriminately in patients whose intracranial pressure is raised, it may have fatal results. It is, of course, necessary when meningitis is suspected, as for instance when there is fever and neck stiffness. It is, however, important to rule out the presence of a haematoma in the first instance. In cases of traumatic subarachnoid haemorrhage, lumbar draining of blood-stained cerebrospinal fluid may help to reduce morbidity and prevent the later development of hydrocephalus.

Lumbar air encephalography

This has all the disadvantages of lumbar puncture and is not used in the management of acute head injuries.

Radioisotope encephalography

The method has been largely superseded by the CT scan, although it still is of some value in centres where the latter is not available. It may be positive in a patient with an intracranial haematoma but it is of limited discriminatory value.

The electroencephalogram

This is used in some intensive therapy units for the diagnosis of irreversible brain death (see below). It does not have a significant part to play in the management of acute head injury but it may be of value in the assessment of patients who are sedated or who have received long-acting paralysing drugs.

CLINICAL DIAGNOSIS OF HAEMATOMA

Intracranial haematoma

Intracranial haematomas compress the brain and in most instances produce coma as the result of rostro-caudal herniation of the brain stem and the supratentorial structures through the tentorial hiatus. A progressive deterioration in the level of consciousness is the most reliable index of increasing intracranial pressure from a haematoma and the importance of serial recordings of the level of consciousness has already been emphasized. Increasing restlessness is an uncommon sign of slowly evolving surface haematoma and is often accompanied by persistent rubbing of the particular area of the scalp over the surface of the position of the clot. The development of a unilateral dilated pupil and increasing hemiparesis may be of particular diagnostic value when previous levels of consciousness have not been diligently noted.

Extradural haematoma

An extradural haematoma is an acute and eminently treatable complication of blunt head injury, though it is relatively rare. With advancing years the dura becomes increasingly adherent to the skull and difficult to separate from the inner table. This is why extradural haematoma is essentially an affliction of youth. More than half of these affected are under the age of 20, and it is a rare condition in people over 40. It is, however, exceptional in infancy, when a blow tends to indent the pliable skull and dura together so that any damage inflicted is borne directly by the brain, and more often the haematoma collects inside the dura mater than outside.

Prognosis is determined by two factors: (1) the severity of the primary brain damage, and (2) the extent to which the secondary disturbance due to distortion of the brain stem has progressed before surgery can be undertaken. In practice, if a patient has been deeply unconscious and unresponsive from the beginning, he is not going to be helped by surgery. If a patient who was reacting briskly and localizing light stimuli on admission has been allowed to deteriorate to a stage where his pupils are widely dilated and he is apnoeic, then death, or at best a persistent vegetative state (see below), is virtually certain.

Subdural haematoma

Unlike the extradural haematoma, the subdural form is an all-too-common complication of head injury with a high mortality and morbidity. The prognosis after an acute subdural haematoma is governed more by the severity of the original impact and the rapidity with which the bleeding has occurred than by the speed and skill with which measures are applied to deal with it. In this respect it differs from the chronic subdural haematoma. Subdural haematomas may be classified into a number of different types.

1   The explosive subdural haematoma usually results from a violent impact. The patient is deeply unconscious from the outset and thence develops signs indicating rostro-caudal herniation with death ensuing within six to twelve hours.

2   The acute subdural haematoma evolves rather more slowly within the first 24 hours and there is often an early period of recovery before deterioration sets in. Mortality is approximately 75% and good recovery is rare.

3   Subacute subdural haematoma typically develops in patients who have shown initial recovery of consciousness and then begin to deteriorate from the second day onwards. Mortality is less than 20%.

4   The chronic subdural haematoma is seen in the elderly and there is often no history of previous head injury.

Investigation of a suspected haematoma

The variety of neuroradiological and other investigations that are available to detect intracranial haematoma in the patient after trauma was considered earlier. The indications for such investigations have already been discussed, but there are also patients in whom intracranial haematomas may be suspected and who need immediate surgery. The following groups of patients should be considered for immediate surgery without recourse to special investigation.

1   The patient is unconscious but is known to have spoken after the injury.
2   The level of consciousness deteriorates noticeably in the course of the initial examination.
3   The patient has developed extensor motor responses in hospital when he was not showing these before admission.
4   The patient is showing extensor motor responses and no history is available.

All of such patients should probably be considered for burr hole exploration.

Cerebral oedema

Professor Brian Jennett from Glasgow coined the phrase 'patients who talk then die' to apply to a group of patients who, following an injury in which they are rendered unconscious for a period of time, then recover and may remain conscious for some hours. Subsequently, the patients deteriorate and, as might have been expected, a proportion of these have intracranial haematomas of one type or another. A significant proportion of these patients, however, have no evidence of intracranial haematoma but simply have cerebral oedema which has resulted from cerebral contusion, laceration, hypoxia or ischaemia. In many rapidly fatal injuries massive cerebral oedema occurs almost immediately after the impact and results from distension of the entire cerebrovascular bed with vasomotor paralysis and failure of normal cerebral autoregulation. Unconsciousness after head injury, however, is *not* always accompanied by such oedema. Typically, cerebral oedema presents clinically with deteriorating consciousness, increasing focal neurological deficit or increasing restlessness. The diagnosis is usually made by appropriate changes on the CT scan or by a negative burr hole exploration. Treatment is unsatisfactory and falls into three main categories: pharmacological, mechanical and surgical.

Treatment of cerebral oedema

Dehydration in one form or other is popular in the management of acute head injury in an attempt to treat cerebral oedema. Mannitol in a dose of 1.5 to 2 g/kg body weight given over a period of 30–60 minutes in a 20–25% solution is perhaps the most widely used agent. Corticosteroids, though used widely, rarely achieve much reduction in pressure in less than 24 hours, and current evidence suggests that these are ineffective, even in very high dosage, in the reduction of intracranial pressure in patients with head injury.

Of all the methods of reducing intracranial pressure the one most readily available and rapid in action is controlled ventilation. Despite its proven efficacy in elective procedures it has not been as widely applied in the management of trauma as some ardent protagonists of the regimen would wish. On the continent of Europe and in the United States there is a tendency to use it much more freely and aggressively than in the United Kingdom, where reluctance probably stems from a fear that such intensive measures may save life at the expense of a persistent vegetative state. When such treatment is instituted, intracranial pressure monitoring should probably be started. Increasingly now, it is agreed among neurosurgeons that the aim should be to start continuous monitoring of intracranial pressure as soon as a haematoma has been ruled out or treated and the presence of a tense swollen brain has been confirmed. The technical details of this are beyond the scope of this chapter.

SPECIFIC PROBLEMS IN PATIENTS AFTER MULTIPLE TRAUMA

The effect of therapy

The problems of the assessment of patients who have received drugs or muscle relaxants have already been considered in brief. If at all possible, such patients should be evaluated before any therapy is given, but this may be impossible. In such instances it may be necessary to perform serial investigations such as echoencephalography or CT scans in order to try to spot the development of an intracranial haematoma. Life-threatening haematomas usually develop within the first few days of injury and serial investigations do not need to be made for longer than this short period. In the later stages, it is usually possible to make neurological investigations when the drugs are beginning to wear off. However, it should always be remembered that the patient after trauma may metabolize such drugs more slowly than the normal healthy individual and allowance should always be made for this.

Prolonged coma

The patient who remains in coma for more than a few days is always a source for concern. The most obvious worry, other than the diagnosis, is whether or not the patient will recover. Unfortunately, medical techniques can assure the survival of many acutely ill comatose patients who never regain apparent psychological awareness. Many of these patients retain sufficient function of their respiratory, cardiovascular, gastrointestinal and urinary systems to sustain a vegetative existence and the term 'vegetative state' was suggested to describe patients who recover the arousal component of consciousness but not awareness. Such patients emerge from coma as evidenced by eye opening and initially this results from stimulation, though eventually occurs spontaneously. Sleep–wake cycles may develop as evidenced by periods of eye opening and eye closure. Brain stem reflexes become brisk and conjugate and dysconjugate roving eye movements may be present. There is, however, no evidence of cognitive activity as evidenced by speech and movement to command. Flaccidity in the limbs may be seen initially though eventually a marked increase in tone develops with increase in the tendon reflexes, extensor plantar responses and appearance of primitive reflexes such as the pouting reflex. This impression of being awake but unaware is a constant source of distress to relatives who find it hard to comprehend that eye opening does not indicate recovery. Persistence of this state for more than a few weeks indicates extensive cortical damage and recovery is most exceptional.

This spectre always haunts the physician who is faced with a patient who remains in coma. In practice, it is important to make a careful assessment of such patients bearing in mind the different problems that are listed in Table 6. The effect of drugs in prolonging apparent coma cannot be overemphasized and this may be readily recognized by the selective effect of such drugs on reflex eye movements. Consideration of prolonged coma and the relationship of this to the vegetative state leads logically to the problem of prediction of outcome in coma.

Prediction of outcome of coma

Until relatively recently little information was available concerning prediction of outcome of patients in coma. Studies funded by the National Institute of Neurological and Communicative Disorders and Stroke have now started to provide such information. There is little doubt that if it were possible to predict a poor outcome for a patient, at an early stage of coma, then those precious intensive therapy facilities which are available would be used more effectively. Conversely, if one were able to identify at an early stage of coma those patients with a reasonable hope of recovery, then more exhaustive attempts at resuscitation and life support would be indicated.

The main determinants of outcome in coma are the cause of the coma, the length and depth of coma and the pattern of the neurological signs of coma.

Aetiology of coma

Coma after trauma may be due to one or more of a variety of causes (Table 6). Where the conscious level is depressed by drugs, then the prognosis is likely to be good. Coma after head injury which persists for more than a few hours is associated with at least a 50% mortality. The patient who is in coma as a result of hypoxic brain damage has a mortality in the region of 60%.

Duration and depth of coma

Not surprisingly, the more prolonged the coma and the deeper the coma the worse the prognosis. For example, the patient who remains in coma for as long as seven days has a 40% chance of remaining in the vegetative state whilst this percentage rises to over 60% if coma persists for two weeks.

Physical signs and outcome

It has now been shown that a variety of physical signs, either in isolation or in combination, may indicate a good or bad prognosis in the patient in coma after trauma.

It is perhaps not surprising that the brain stem reflexes provide significant prognostic information, particularly in the prediction of poor outcome. More specific information concerning prediction of outcome in this situation may be found in the references to this chapter.

Recently there has been some interest in the value of neurophysiological investigation in estimating prognosis in coma. Certain patterns of abnormality on conventional encephalography are associated with poor prognosis, and prolonged EEG recording with computer analysis has been suggested as a predictor of outcome equal to clinical assessment. More sophisticated electrophysiological techniques, such as auditory evoked responses and blink reflexes, have also been suggested as useful predictors of outcome.

BRAIN DEATH

The 1980 BBC television programme 'Panorama' concerning brain death provoked a widespread controversy concerning the reliability of the United Kingdom brain death criteria. This controversy resulted in part from ignorance concerning the United Kingdom criteria (Table 8) and partly from differing interpretations of the term 'brain death'.

Table 8. The diagnosis of brain death: United Kingdom criteria

---

1. Conditions under which the diagnosis of brain death should be considered:
   (a) The patient is deeply comatose
      (i) There should be no suspicion that this state is due to depressant drugs
      (ii) Primary hypothermia as a cause of coma should have been excluded
      (iii) Metabolic and endocrine disturbances which can be responsible for or can contribute to coma should have been excluded
   (b) The patient is being maintained on a ventilator because spontaneous respiration had previously become inadequate or had ceased altogether. Relaxants (neuromuscular blocking agents) and other drugs should have been excluded as a cause of respiratory inadequacy or failure
   (c) There should be no doubt that the patient's condition is due to irremediable structural brain damage. The diagnosis of a disorder which can lead to brain death should have been fully established

2. Diagnostic tests for the confirmation of brain death:
   All brainstem reflexes are absent:
   (a) The pupils are fixed in diameter and do not respond to sharp changes in the intensity of incident light
   (b) There is no corneal reflex
   (c) The vestibulo-ocular reflexes are absent
   (d) No motor responses within the cranial nerve distribution can be elicited by adequate stimulation of any somatic area
   (e) There is no gag reflex or reflex responses to bronchial stimulation by a suction catheter passed down the trachea
   (f) No respiratory movements occur when the patient is disconnected from the mechanical ventilator for long enough to ensure that the arterial carbon dioxide tension rises above the threshold for stimulation of respiration

---

The criteria may be simply stated as:
1 Irremedial structural brain damage
2 Apnoeic coma not due to drugs, hypothermia or a metabolic disturbance
3 Absent brain reflexes
4 No cranial nerve motor responses, no gag reflex and no respiratory movement on disconnection of ventilator ($Pa\text{CO}_2$ to rise above 6.8 kPa)

It is confidently believed in the United Kingdom that all such patients will die and the examples shown in the television programme did not fulfil the strict criteria. In the United States a variety of criteria has been described, and the most recent have been endorsed by the American Academy of Neurology Executive Committee. The clinical criteria are similar to the United Kingdom criteria, though it is suggested that the diagnosis should not be applied in children under five years of age, and it is recommended that 'confirmation of clinical findings by EEG' is desirable.

Brain death and electroencephalogram

Because the diagnosis of brain death carries such a heavy clinical and legal responsibility, many regard additional laboratory investigations as essential. The EEG is the most widely used and it is generally accepted that an isoelectric EEG for 12 hours in a patient with structural brain damage indicates that no chance of recovery exists. In America a national cooperative group has published the technical requirements necessary to establish electrocerebral silence. The need for investigations other than EEG is controversial, but it has been suggested that the high organ donation rate in Norway has resulted from public confidence in their brain death criteria which includes four vessel cerebral angiography and requires radiographic absence of the cerebral circulation. The risks of this are obvious and other safer techniques for studying cerebral circulation, such as radionuclide scintography and common carotid doppler velographic tracings, are at present being tested.

Because of differing attitudes to brain death the term itself has been criticized and it has been suggested that it should be abandoned. However, with few exceptions there is general agreement that the brain and the person are one and hence a patient who fills the criteria can be regarded as *dead*. The issue of organ donation is separate as this involves the patient's or family's wishes. The timing of organ removal in relation to discontinuation of treatment is another controversial area with differing practices, though the decision to discontinue support should be undertaken only with the informed consent of relatives or guardian. A code of practice for the removal of cadaveric organs for transplantation has been published in the United Kingdom on behalf of the Health Department of Great Britain and Northern Ireland.

THE USE OF SEDATIVE/HYPNOTIC DRUGS IN THE TREATMENT OF SEVERE BRAIN INJURY

In addition to the methods of treatment mentioned above—diuretics, corticosteroids, hyperventilation—barbiturates (usually thiopentone or pentabarbitone) or Althesin (alphaxalone–alphadolone acetate) are widely used. Although this type of treatment has been tried sporadically in the past its systemic use has a shorter provenance. The objectives of treatment include reduction of cerebral metabolic rate, reduction of intracranial pressure, and abolition of epileptic convulsions.

Thiopentone is more reliable than Althesin for these purposes and is usually given as an initial dose of 1 g/h, gradually reducing to 350–500 mg/h by continuous infusion. Althesin is given initially at 10 ml/h. Both regimens may be monitored either by direct measurement of intracranial pressure or with the cerebral function monitor. The primary objective is to reduce intracranial pressure to below 25 mmHg; cerebral electrical activity should also be suppressed.

Many clinicians prefer Althesin to thiopentone because of its shorter half-life. Patients given thiopentone by infusion for more than 48 hours cannot be expected to recover their pre-infusion activity within less than 24 hours. However, thiopentone is a more effective anticonvulsant than Althesin.

Early publications suggested that this treatment had revolutionized the prognosis for brain-damaged patients, but measured assessment has resulted in a more cautious estimation of its value.

The patient always requires endotracheal intubation to protect his airway; he usually receives controlled hyperventilation and may also be given corticosteroids, in spite of the evidence which suggests them to be valueless. Mannitol and other diuretic agents are also commonly used. Because they are usually given in combination therapy, the value of barbiturates or Althesin cannot be adequately assessed; it is probable that any benefit they confer is marginal.

Neuromuscular blocking agents must not be used as the sole means of suppressing epileptic convulsions; there is evidence which suggests that the abolition of muscular activity without simultaneous suppression of cerebral seizure activity increases the likelihood of permanent cerebral damage.

References

Department of Health and Social Security (1979) *The Removal of Cadaveric Organs for Transplantation: A Code of Practice*. London: HMSO.

Jennett, B. & Teasdale, G. (1981) *Management of Head Injuries*. 361 pp. Philadelphia: F.A. Davis.

Levy, D.E., Bates, D., Caronna, J. et al (1981) Prognosis in non-traumatic coma. *Annals of Internal Medicine*, **94**, 293–301.

Marshall, L.F., Smith, R.W. & Shapiro, H.M. (1979) The outcome with aggressive treatment in severe head injuries. *Journal of Neurosurgery*, **56**, 26–30.

Miller, J.D. (1979) Barbiturates and raised intracranial pressure. *Annals of Neurology*, **6**(3), 189–193.

Moss, E., Gibson, J.S., McDowell, D.G. & Gibson, R.M. (1983) Intensive management of severe head injuries. *Anaesthesia*, **38**(3), 214–225.

Plum, F. & Posner, J.B. (1980) *The Diagnosis of Stupor and Coma*. Third Edition. 373 pp. Philadelphia: F.A. Davis.

Safar, P., Bleyaert, A., Nemoto, E.M. et al (1978) Resuscitation after global brain ischaemia/anoxia. *Critical Care Medicine*, **6**, 215–227.

Vinken, P.J. & Bruyn, G.W. (1975) Injuries of the brain and skull; Parts I and II. *Handbook of Clinical Neurology*, Volumes **23** and **24**. Amsterdam, New York: Elsevier North-Holland.

9

Hypothermia, Exposure, Drowning

These three conditions have one notable feature in common, namely, a subnormal body temperature. Hypothermia is defined as a core temperature of 35°C or below, although usually the only result of this degree of cooling is discomfort and shivering. The lowest body temperature which is compatible with survival after accidental exposure is uncertain, since many anecdotal and improbable figures are quoted and because it is so difficult to measure core temperature in the field. However, a wealth of data support the following generalizations:

Below 33°C—shivering may cease and consciousness becomes clouded.
Below 30°C—consciousness is lost and cardiac dysrhythmias appear.
Below 28°C—the 'fibrillation threshold': ventricular fibrillation is common.
Below 27°C—life is difficult to detect without an ECG; the EEG may be flat, the pupils dilate, the patient is areflexic.
Below 25°C—cardiac arrest may occur.

It must be realized, however, that prolonged survival and successful resuscitation have been recorded when the core temperature has been below 25°C, and resuscitation attempts should not be abandoned until the patient has been re-warmed. The appropriate aphorism is: 'nobody is dead until he is warm and dead'.

When the core temperature reaches 28°C the metabolic oxygen consumption is halved and, provided the extremities are protected from circulatory stasis, recovery may be uneventful. At least one patient is known to have survived after spending the night unconscious in a snowdrift; when found, her core temperature was 15°C.

Measurement of body temperature

The oral and axillary routes are useless when the patient is really cold, and the fact that the oral temperature is so unreliable is probably responsible for the misleadingly high incidence of accidental hypothermia in the elderly which is reported each winter. The oral temperature falls rapidly during mouth breathing in a cold environment and the axillary temperature is influenced by vasoconstriction and a lowered cardiac output. However, there is little doubt that the diagnosis is often missed, particularly since the range of the standard clinical thermometer is 35–43°C. The range of the low-reading thermometer is 30–40°C and there is little justification for continuing to use the standard clinical thermometer in a country which has a climate which is classified as 'north-temperate and bracing', which has innumerable rivers and hills and which is entirely surrounded by water with a temperature which ranges between 2 and 10°C. Even in tropical regions the sea water temperature is such that hypothermia may follow prolonged partial immersion provided the victim survives the attention of sharks, rays and electric eels.

There are several alternative sites from which to record the core temperature since the objectives are to measure the temperature of the brain and the heart. The temperature of arterial blood most closely represents the true core temperature, but is not routinely measured. The temperature measured in the occluded external auditory canal approximates to brain temperature; an oesophageal probe with its tip 24 cm from the teeth or gums gives a close approximation to heart temperature and is not affected by respiratory gas movement in the trachea. Rectal thermometry is less satisfactory, both because at present it is socially unacceptable to the conscious adult and because its readings are 'damped' by faeces so that it lags behind the rapidly changing true core temperature by an important amount. The temperature in the nasopharynx is close to that of the hypothalamus but it is difficult to position the probe securely and it is subject to respiratory artefact.

In domiciliary practice none of these methods is fully acceptable. It is said that the temperature of freshly voided urine gives a good indication of deep body temperature but this technique is rarely practicable in the home. As with many other conditions in medicine, a high index of suspicion is necessary. Any patient who is cold to the touch but is not complaining of the cold or shivering should be considered to be at risk.

Accidental hypothermia

The body temperature is maintained at 37 ± 0.2°C, the upper level being recorded at approximately 4 p.m. It is controlled by the anterior hypothalamus which appears to have a temperature set point such that variations outside this range activate homeostatic mechanisms. The body generates heat by increasing the metabolic rate, shivering, non-shivering thermogenesis in brown fat, and by releasing metabolically active hormones which include growth hormone, thyroxine and noradrenaline.

Contributory causes

Heat regulation is disturbed in circumstances which include:
1   The extremes of age
2   The presence of conditions such as hypopituitarism, diabetes, Addison's disease, myxoedema, and infective illnesses, particularly pneumonia
3   Coma due to cerebral vascular accidents, head injuries, uraemia, or hepatic failure
4   General anaesthesia and other drugs, including alcohol, antidepressants, antihistamines, barbiturates, benzodiazepines, and phenothiazines

Beta blocking drugs prevent heat being generated in brown fat; several patients with subclinical myxoedema who have received drugs of this type for the treatment of cardiac dysrhythmias have become hypothermic.

Hypothermia which originates in the operating room is discussed later.

The effects of ageing

Most patients who are found to have a subnormal body temperature are suffering from one of the conditions listed, but the elderly, frail, self-neglectful or indigent patient is particularly at risk in cold weather. There is evidence which suggests that the elderly patient, particularly if he is suffering from some chronic debilitating disease, is not so aware of the cold as a fit, younger person and therefore does not take precautions to keep warm. Many elderly patients are afraid to heat their homes because of the cost, in spite of the fact that this can usually be defrayed by the local authorities.

A surprising number of elderly people drink large amounts of alcohol, and this has been the principal contributory factor in most of the patients seen by the author. Alcohol depresses the hypothalamus, causes peripheral vasodilatation, and predisposes to falls, injury and unconsciousness.

There is evidence that even in the absence of overt endocrine abnormalities such as myxoedema and Addison's disease, elderly patients have a subnormal metabolic rate. The average body heat production of patients who are between 20 and 40 years of age is $155 \text{ kJ}/\text{m}^2/\text{h}$ whereas that of patients over 60 years of age is reduced to an average of $128 \text{ kJ}/\text{m}^2/\text{h}$. Diabetes is occasionally associated with dysautonomia. This can be recognized from the ECG rhythm strip by measuring the T–T interval during several respiratory cycles. The normal sinus arrhythmia is absent in the patient with dysautonomia and such a patient is at great risk of hypothermia in cold weather.

Any patient who has such advanced cardiocirculatory disease that he is unable to respond to a demand for an increased cardiac output is in danger of hypothermia both directly and because this tends to encourage immobility.

ACCIDENTAL HYPOTHERMIA AND GENERAL ANAESTHESIA

Anaesthetists have become increasingly aware of the fact that patients usually cool while undergoing general anaesthesia and a small proportion become very cold indeed. This can occur in association with any surgical procedure, but it is particularly common in patients who are undergoing prolonged neurosurgical, orthopaedic and major vascular surgery (e.g. aortofemoral bypass). It is very likely to occur in patients who are receiving emergency treatment for extensive burns because of evaporative heat losses. There is evidence which suggests that burned tissue releases a substance which interferes with hypothalamic temperature control. Patients with high cervical cord injury which results in cervico-dorsal sympathectomy may also become hypothermic.

Although the duration of the operative procedure is important, most of the cooling occurs during the first 60 minutes of anaesthesia and surgery. The core temperature is commonly found to range between 33°C and 35°C, whereas the skin temperature, measured on the dorsum of the hand or foot, may be as low as 20°C and if measured on the toes or fingers, correspondingly lower.

Effect of anaesthetic agents

Many of the contributory factors have already been mentioned. They include the fact that elderly patients have a diminished heat production which is aggravated by all depressant drugs, which obviously include anaesthetic agents. Approximately 4% of patients over the age of 65 years have a subnormal body temperature on admission to hospital in the winter months and this number is increased to 10% after the pre-anaesthetic medication is given.

General anaesthesia induces a poikilothermic state so that the protective vasoconstriction and shivering which should occur when a patient is exposed to the cool operating room environment are abolished. The additional effect of neuromuscular blockade is probably unimportant, although it is possible that the spontaneously breathing patient generates a small amount of heat in his respiratory muscles.

Environmental cooling

When the gut is exposed to a cold environment, or when wet packs or wet drapes are applied, heat loss accelerates in proportion to the rate of water evaporation (2.5 kJ/g water). The thermal conductivity of water is 30 times greater than that of air. This fact has greater relevance for those patients suffering from exposure or near-drowning, but it is also important in the operating room. The scalp has a very rich blood supply, and the amount of heat lost from the unprotected head, particularly if it is largely hairless, represents an important fraction of the total heat produced by the anaesthetized or unconscious patient. There may also be a significant loss of heat through evaporation of water from the respiratory tract. This has been calculated to be up to 40 kJ/h for adults ventilated with dry gases at 10 l/min. Blood transfused straight from the refrigerator may add to the cooling effect; it has been stated that blood at 4°C will reduce the core temperature by 1°C per litre infused although this figure is almost certainly an overestimate.

When the aortic clamp is applied during major vascular surgery, the lower half of the body cools more rapidly than the upper, so that when the clamp is removed cold blood is flushed from the lower limbs and the blood which perfuses them cools further.

Although these factors may play a part, by far the most important cause of hypothermia is the ambient temperature; it has been shown that providing this is maintained above 21°C no significant cooling occurs during routine surgery without excessive evaporative losses. If the ambient temperature is greater than 24°C the patient is in danger of hyperpyrexia.

Unfortunately, but understandably, many surgeons prefer to work in a cool environment; however, there is no doubt that it is more important for the surgeon to be comfortable than for the patient to be exposed to an environmental temperature which is theoretically ideal.

The consequences of accidental hypothermia

These are directly related to the extent of the drop in temperature, and patients with moderately severe hypothermia (core temperature 31–34°C) may have no long-lasting effects. If the core temperature falls below this more serious problems can arise, but it is most important to avoid over-reaction to metabolic disturbances which will correct themselves as the patient re-warms.

The metabolic effects of hypothermia

These include:

1   Fluid redistribution resulting in increased central blood volume, increased haematocrit and increased blood viscosity

2   Non-respiratory acidaemia and/or lactic acidaemia, particularly if the patient is allowed to shiver

3   Disseminated intravascular coagulation—this is rarely important clinically at core temperatures greater than 31°C

4   Depressed liver function—which may prolong drug effects and give rise to shortage of coagulation factors

5   Glucose intolerance due to diminished uptake, reduced insulin production and catecholamine secretion

6   Hypertension due to vasoconstriction and catecholamine secretion

7   Cold diuresis—this may occasionally be mistaken for acute tubular necrosis and accentuates the loss of circulating blood volume

Provided that the cause of these disturbances is recognized the attendant can concentrate his attention on warming the patient safely and can almost ignore the metabolic effects.

Hypothermia causes prolonged peripheral vasoconstriction which is followed by loss of plasma water into the tissues. The increased central blood volume encourages a diuresis which is augmented by the effect of cold blood on the kidneys. Therefore, as the patient warms he will require infusion of saline and plasma protein fraction to refill the capacitance vessels and the peripheral circulation.

The effects of cooling upon hydrogen ion status

The effects of cooling upon hydrogen ion status are very complex. As the body cools, the production of hydrogen ions and carbon dioxide is reduced, but if the tissue perfusion falls before the metabolic rate falls, excess hydrogen ions in the form of carbonic and lactic acid are generated. This difficulty is compounded by two other problems. In the first place it is known that as the body cools the pH of neutrality rises, and a pH which is alkaline at normal body temperature is acidic at a lower temperature. The other problem concerns the need to measure blood gases and pH at the temperature at which the blood was sampled. Any non-respiratory hydrogen ion abnormality must be corrected cautiously and minimally if at all; otherwise, as the patient reaches normal body temperature it will be found to have been overcorrected and the patient will have a very marked non-respiratory alkalaemia which may need to be corrected in turn. For the same reason, hyperglycaemia and glycosuria should not be treated until the patient has regained the normal body temperature.

The clinical consequences of hypothermia

The greatest danger for the patient who has cooled during major surgery is that the changes which occur during re-warming are mistaken for internal bleeding. When he arrives in the ITU or surgical ward, his blood pressure is usually raised above the pre-anaesthetic level (Figure 21). As he re-warms, the resulting vasodilatation causes the blood pressure to fall, sometimes dramatically, while the pulse rate rises. The central venous pressure also falls. Unless the patient's core and skin temperature have been noted on return from theatre, these signs are liable to be misinterpreted and the patient submitted to an unnecessary and potentially hazardous re-operation.

If the cause is recognized, the patient should be given a blood volume expander such as Haemaccel at a carefully regulated rate while his hourly

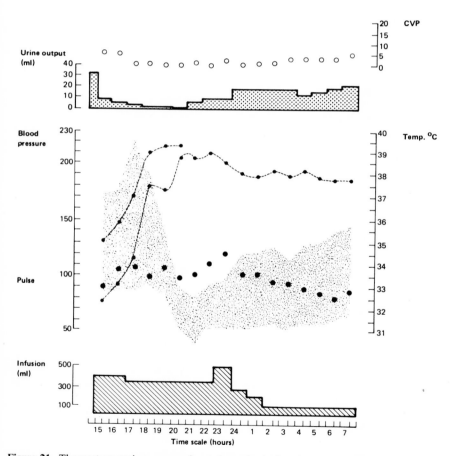

Figure 21. The post-operative course of a patient who had undergone three hours of arterial surgery. The lightly stippled area in the centre demonstrates the changes in blood pressure which occurred.

urine volume output and its osmolality are recorded. The danger of overtransfusion and pulmonary oedema are particularly acute in the re-warming patient. If the patient has undergone major vascular surgery, the pulses and temperature of his lower limbs must be monitored at frequent short intervals to exclude the possibility of obstruction or leakage at the anastomotic site.

Acute pancreatitis

This complication of hypothermia has been reported on many occasions and it may have contributed to the death of several patients. It is believed that hypothermia causes pancreatic arterial vasoconstriction, while thrombosis and intravascular coagulation may also play a part. The condition may not be obvious since many other events occur simultaneously, and the serum amylase must be measured every 24 hours in the hypothermic patient and after rewarming.

EXPOSURE

Exposure is a more dramatic and usually more obvious form of accidental hypothermia which may be aggravated by the signs of peripheral vascular injury such as frostbite, which is the result of sustained vasoconstriction, intravascular thrombosis and external moist cooling. Most of the patients who are suffering from exposure are either in occupations for which the condition is a recognized hazard (fishermen, seamen, shepherds, military personnel) or have chosen to pit their abilities against a hostile environment for recreational purposes (climbers, walkers, potholers). In general these patients are in a younger age group than those who suffer from accidental hypothermia and many of them are athletic and physically fit. Nevertheless, the mortality rate from the condition is considerable, and in the United Kingdom at least 20 persons per year die from exposure on the land, and an unknown number die at sea from the same cause but are usually said to have drowned. Near-drowning is discussed on page 160.

Contributory factors

The most important contributory factors include the use of unsuitable clothing together with a change in the weather and an unforeseen emergency. The combination of a low environmental temperature, high wind and wet garments inevitably causes a rapid loss of body heat (the wind chill factor). Persons who are particularly at risk are those who have allowed themselves to become exhausted.

If the victim is misguidedly persuaded to remain active, that is, 'to walk about to keep warm', particularly if he sweats or is wearing wet clothing, he will lose heat much more rapidly than if he lies at rest in the lea of any available shelter, preferably wearing dry clothing supplied by his colleagues. In the open air, shivering and exercise accelerate heat loss and precipitate death from hypothermia.

At low ambient temperatures the heat lost from the respiratory tract may exceed the body's total heat production. Fishermen sitting in small open boats are exposed to the additional hazard of the 'heat sink' through the poorly insulated hull.

All of the factors listed earlier as causes of hypothermia may contribute. Alcohol is the principal drug taken by the exposure victim, often for its 'warming' properties, although it invariably accelerates the cooling process.

The prevention and treatment of accidental hypothermia and exposure

A knowledge of the factors that cause heat loss allows preventative measures to be practised in the operating room. These include the maintenance of a warm environment and the avoidance of draughts, which include those from air-conditioning inlets. The limitation placed upon this recommendation by the surgeon's preference has been mentioned.

A heated humidifier, a warming mattress and infusion warming devices should be routinely used during prolonged operative procedures. For safety, all heated humidifiers must be fitted with a thermostatic alarm. Although they may be capable of producing only 75–85% humidification they effectively prevent heat loss from the respiratory tract. Several cases have been reported in which patients have suffered skin burns from water mattresses heated to 40°C, particularly during the course of vascular operations. These are due to the fact that ischaemic tissues have a lower thermal capacity than tissues with a good blood supply. Very few infusion warmers can warm to 37°C more than 3.0 litres of banked blood per hour.

Prevention of evaporative losses

The avoidance or limitation of gut exposure and wet packs depends upon surgical skills, speed and technique, but the anaesthetist must not hesitate to tell the surgeon if an unnecessarily large amount of gut is exposed, or is covered with a warm wet pack which has cooled down.

The prevention of evaporative and convective cooling of other parts of the body—particularly the head, shoulders and chest—is very important. These areas should be covered with heat-insulating material, and 'space blankets' are commonly used. Several investigators have shown that this material is no better than conventional cellular blankets for this purpose, but it is very easy to handle and clean. However, if it is not tucked in firmly around the patient, draughts can easily get at him.

Post-operative care

When the patient returns to the ITU or ward, these measures should be continued, and in particular the patient's cubicle or bed area should be warm and draught free. Occasionally the patient's skin temperature does not rise quickly and it may be necessary to apply pharmacological assistance, but this is done only if the patient's blood volume is known to be adequate. Peripheral cooling and vasoconstriction are usually due to the combined effects of cooling and hypovolaemia; a warm environment and blood volume replacement are the only treatment required. The indications for the use of vasodilator drugs are exactly the same as those described in Chapter 2, namely, a wide core-to-skin temperature difference, often accompanied by visible evidence of poor skin perfusion (pallor, peripheral cyanosis), a high or normal blood pressure and a high central venous pressure. If these criteria are met the patient should be given chlorpromazine 12.5 mg intravenously, repeated if necessary after 30 minutes. Rarely, this is followed by a marked drop in blood pressure, which is an indication for increasing the rate of volume replacement. The choice of fluid for this purpose has been discussed in Chapter 2.

Pyrexial overshoot

Patients who are cold on return from the operating room almost invariably show a pyrexial overshoot two to four hours later, and this is often mistaken for a transfusion reaction or septicaemia (Figure 21). It is a sensible precaution to take a blood culture at this stage but nothing else need be done since the temperature usually returns to normal within a few hours. The elevated temperature is often accompanied by hypotension which responds to further fluid infusion, but it is essential not to be tempted into the danger of overtransfusion since many of these patients are in danger of renal impairment, pulmonary oedema, or ARDS.

The treatment of severe hypothermia

Severe hypothermia is defined either as hypothermia which is not responding satisfactorily to standard methods of treatment, or as a core temperature below 32°C. In most cases it is caused by exposure either in the home or in the open air together with one or more of the predisposing factors listed earlier.

Treatment in the field

Wherever possible the patient should be transferred to the ITU of the nearest hospital for treatment, but he must be handled very gently since rough handling has been known to cause circulatory failure and fatal dysrhythmias. In the field, only limited treatment is available. This includes removal of wet clothing and its replacement with dry blankets. The space blanket tends to flap and it should itself be surrounded by another blanket—or, even better, the patient should be placed inside a sleeping bag. Cold extremities should not be 'massaged' or exposed to local heating, since massage may occasionally cause a further drop in core temperature, as the cold blood leaves the periphery and re-enters the central circulation. Local heat may burn the poorly perfused skin.

Warming of inspired air Airway warming is widely recommended, and even if it does not actually provide much heat, it does prevent the patient losing further heat through evaporation of water vapour from the respiratory tract. The principle is exactly the same as that of the 'Waters canister' carbon dioxide absorber, and many rescue services use this system. As the patient breathes out, his expired air and carbon dioxide warm the soda line so that the next inspired breath is warmed and partly humidified. Since very cold patients produce little carbon dioxide, a modification is available which allows carbon dioxide from a sparklet cylinder to pre-warm the soda line. The canister is usually insulated in a woollen bag or similar device. The face mask must be closely applied to the victim's face since any leakage of cold air rapidly neutralizes the beneficial effects of the canister. Alternative methods using mouthpieces have been tried with varying degrees of success.

Treatment in hospital

After the patient arrives in hospital more active methods of re-warming may be used. As with other types of hypothermia, a warm environment and minimum exposure are essential.

Controlled ventilation Most patients who are suffering from moderate or severe hypothermia benefit from controlled ventilation with oxygen-enriched, warmed, humidified air, and endotracheal intubation should prevent asphyxia or aspiration of secretions and vomit. However, the effects of hypothermia upon metabolic rate have already been referred to and overventilation must be avoided. Moderate hypoventilation is safer than hyperventilation, particularly since carbon dioxide accumulation encourages systemic and pulmonary vasodilatation and shifts the haemoglobin dissociation curve to the right. Hypothermia has minimal effects upon carbon dioxide carriage, and provided that the measurements are made at the temperature at which the specimens were taken, the results are meaningful.

Active re-warming If the patient is otherwise well and re-warming spontaneously there is no need to use active re-warming methods, although several are available. The simplest and in many ways the best is to immerse the patient in water at 40°C until his core temperature has reached 33°C, at which temperature active re-warming can be discontinued. A radiant heat cradle can also be used to accelerate the rate of warming although this may cause blistering. Theoretically there is the danger that external warming will allow blood to perfuse dilated but cold areas and cause further core cooling (the afterdrop), and this has been advanced to explain the occasional sudden death which occurs during and after re-warming. The core and skin temperature must be continuously monitored whichever method of re-warming is used.

Extracorporeal warming Other methods use some form of extracorporeal warming system. If the facilities exist, the heat-exchanger of an extracorporeal oxygenator can be used although this may demand arterial cannulation. The author uses veno-venous dialysis to warm patients whose core temperature is below 31°C if they are not warming steadily (1°C per hour) with non-invasive methods. This has the additional benefit of removing alcohol and some other drugs from the patient's body. Either method of extracorporeal warming has the advantage over external methods that it warms the core in parallel with the periphery.

Prognosis

Whichever method of re-warming is used, the results depend upon the cause. Young or otherwise fit patients usually do well, as do those patients who are hypothermic as a result of coma due to alcohol or drugs. On the other hand, elderly patients who are arteriopathic or diabetic, or who have an infective illness as the precipitating cause, do less well. The cause of death in some cases is not obvious and the author has seen one patient who was allowed to warm gradually from a core temperature of 31°C and who died suddenly when fully conscious at 36°C. No cause was found at autopsy or in the biochemistry laboratory.

DROWNING

This section should really be entitled 'near-drowning' since drowning means death. However, resuscitation is so frequently successful, even in the most apparently hopeless situation, that this term will be retained. In the United Kingdom there are at least 700 deaths from drowning per year, and an unknown number of patients are resuscitated after immersion incidents. In the USA drowning is the third most common cause of accidental death, and in Australia many hundreds of cases are reported annually. In both countries, the private swimming pool is the commonest site of the accident.

Classification of immersion incidents

Immersion incidents are usually divided into salt-water and fresh-water drowning but the effects are not mutually exclusive, and although the classical effects of the two accidents are discussed below, functionally there is very little difference between them. Although pollution is being reduced, most of the major waterways of Britain and other industrialized nations are little better than open sewers. Immersion in this effluent could not by any stretch of the imagination be classed as fresh-water drowning. Even private and municipal swimming pools have a high bacterial, fungal and chemical pollutant level. Sea water close to heavily polluted areas is also often polluted with sewage and the debris from rivers and harbours.

Patients are occasionally seen following immersion in more exotic fluids. The author has recently looked after a 16-month-old child who was found cyanosed and unconscious floating in a 90-litre tub of home-brewed beer. Happily, she made an uneventful recovery in spite of having two hypoxic fits and quite severe respiratory dysfunction. The yeast in the brew caused no specific pulmonary problem.

The effects of immersion

The effects of all forms of immersion are ultimately the same, and many of the observations which are said to distinguish between salt- and fresh-water drowning relate to experiments performed upon animals which bear no direct comparison with the human survivors of near-drowning. Some of the biochemical data which follow are inevitably in this category, but the discussion which follows is based upon clinical experience.

The effects of near-drowning can be considered under the following headings:

1 Asphyxia
2 Biochemical effects
3 Alveolar damage
4 The presence of foreign material
5 Hypothermia
6 Miscellaneous problems

Dry drowning

It is generally stated that up to 10% of all patients who die from drowning do so without having inhaled fluid—the so-called 'dry drowning'. The cause of death in these cases is thought to be either vagal inhibition due to laryngeal stimulation, or acute cardiac failure due to asphyxia in patients with pre-existing severe cardiac disease or hypertension. Cold-water immersion causes an immediate increase in heart rate and blood pressure which may be greater than the diseased cardiocirculatory system can tolerate.

The diving reflex

It is possible that the diving reflex may be involved in dry drowning. This mechanism is well developed in whales and similar mammals and may be present in infants and older humans. When the animal dives there is an immediate slowing of the pulse rate and redistribution of blood from the periphery to the core so that only the vital tissues are perfused. The peripheral tissues cool very rapidly. It has been postulated that death from asystole and hypoxia occurs before the patient inhales a significant amount of fluid into the lungs. After death, water spills over into the tracheobronchial tree. In infants, the reflex is thought to be activated via the trigeminal nerve when the face is immersed in cold water.

Hyperventilation

Cold water immersion causes hyperventilation, and a very low arterial carbon dioxide tension can be achieved. It has been associated with death in competitive swimmers, who sometimes hyperventilate deliberately before diving into the water. They are thought to die from hypoxia before the arterial carbon dioxide tension level is high enough to stimulate breathing.

Pressure effects

Another factor which has been invoked is the pressure effect of the water surrounding the victim as he is immersed. This can cause an increase in venous return in a manner analogous to the 'G-suit', and it has been suggested that some of the victims who die shortly after removal from the water do so because of removal of this effect coupled with vasodilatation due to external warming.

Asphyxia

Although each of these mechanisms may be important there is no doubt that the cause of death in most cases of drowning is asphyxia, with hypothermia in a close second place.

Biochemical effects of drowning

The most obvious biochemical effects are hypoxia and hypercapnia due to asphyxia, followed by acidaemia which results from anaerobic metabolism. The initial effects of fresh-water (hypotonic) and salt-water (hypertonic) immersion have been extensively investigated both in animals and in humans. It is usually stated that the asphyxial effects of sea water are more marked because it causes acute laryngospasm and proteinaceous pulmonary oedema. The other contrasting effects upon the lungs and the blood are related to their constituents which are listed below and illustrated in Figure 22.

Fresh water	*Salt water*
Hypotonic fluid	Hypertonic fluid
Detergents	Sodium
Sewage	Potassium
Solid detritus	Calcium
Organic and inorganic chemicals	Magnesium
	Silica (sand)
	Diatoms etc.
	Contaminants

Since the alveolar membrane is semipermeable the effects of immersion in these solutions should be predictable.

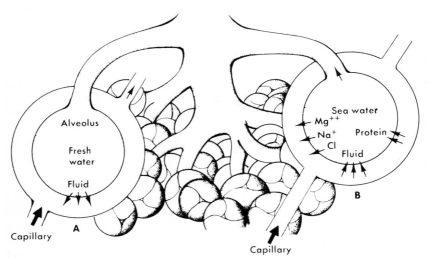

Figure 22. The pulmonary effects of fresh-water (A) and salt-water (B) immersion.

Fresh water is rapidly absorbed, and if a large enough volume is inhaled it causes haemodilution and hyponatraemia. Dilution leads to haemolysis and the serum potassium may rise significantly. In animal experiments, death following fresh-water immersion may be due to asphyxia or to either massive haemolysis or hyperkalaemia.

When salt water reaches the alveoli it must first equilibrate with the extracellular fluid before it can be absorbed and it thereby causes haemoconcentration. After equilibration it is absorbed and its effects include crenation and fragmentation of red cells together with hypernatraemia and hypermagnesaemia.

In either case red cell damage causes hyperkalaemia, although this is said to be more marked immediately after fresh-water immersion. However, clinical experience suggests that by the time they reach hospital most of the survivors of immersion incidents show no obvious differences in serum electrolytes or osmolality.

The effects upon the alveoli

Published data concerning the effects of hypertonic and hypotonic immersion upon the alveolar membrane is inconsistent, and each has been said to be more likely than the other to wash away surfactant and damage the underlying cells.

In the author's experience patients who survive either fresh-water or salt-water drowning have few lasting pulmonary sequelae, provided that the water is reasonably clean. On admission to hospital they are always hypoxic with a wide Aa gradient and have diffuse pulmonary opacities which are more marked around the hilar areas. They may cough up moderate quantities of frothy sputum, and if the patient is clinically dead on arrival, the airway is sometimes full of water, which should be removed by posture or suction. The Aa gradient narrows over the succeeding 24–36 hours, although the radiological abnormalities usually take longer to resolve. After two to four days lung function returns to normal, provided that the lungs have not become infected during the course of treatment.

Immersion in contaminated water

Patients who have been immersed in industrial rivers, or in the sea close to a river mouth, have a quite different course although the initial presentation is similar to that described above. After resuscitation they usually remain hypoxic even on 100% oxygen with PEEP and frequently die several days later with signs of widespread infective pneumonia, often with abscess formation.

All too frequently infants drown in bath-tub water. This has the same effect as clean fresh water although, theoretically, soap-suds can damage the alveolar membrane. After this type of incident, the possibility of non-accidental injury must be considered. One of the author's patients who was admitted after such an incident had cigarette burns on the buttocks and petechial spots over the face and upper chest—the 'Tardieu' spots which are usually seen after manual strangulation.

It must be concluded that the most important features of near-drowning are not the type of fluid the patient is immersed in but its asphyxial effects upon the brain and the contaminants it contains.

Secondary drowning

This is the name given to the sequence in which acute pulmonary oedema with pink frothy sputum, dyspnoea and hypoxia appear 15 minutes to 72 hours after the initial incident. It is equally common after salt-water or fresh-water immersion and may cause death from hypoxia in patients thought to be recovering. It should be distinguished from acute bacterial pneumonia which may present a similar radiographic picture. The treatment of this condition is discussed later.

Very rarely, patients who are either conscious when rescued or who have subsequently regained consciousness lapse into coma with signs of increased intracranial pressure. This may be due to a head injury, but it has also been attributed to secondary cerebral oedema and the outcome is said to be poor.

Hypothermia in near-drowning

The contribution made by hypothermia to death or survival after immersion incidents has been widely discussed. In the first place, because most patients who are removed from the sea or from rivers are cold, it is commonly stated that hypothermia is an important cause of death. Other investigators believe that hypothermia is important only if the patient is prevented from drowning by a lifejacket, and even in these circumstances most victims drown because they lose consciousness and are unable to protect their air passages.

On the credit side, several case reports have been published in which the survival of patients after drowning has been attributed to the fact that they have fallen into very cold water (usually glacial streams or through ice into lakes) and have thereby been protected by the rapid onset of deep hypothermia. All incidents of this kind have concerned small children in whom the ratio surface area/body weight is greater than in the adult. This makes the cooling process much more rapid.

The cardiocirculatory effects of hypothermia have already been discussed. In addition to these, cold immersion invariably causes hyperventilation which may lead to tetany and inability to swim or call for help; even good swimmers are unable to swim for long in very cold water, but in neither of these instances is core hypothermia the critical factor. The duration of immersion and the temperature of the water are both vitally important; rivers and lakes are appreciably warmer than the North Sea in winter. If the victim is wearing a wet suit or other protective clothing he will be able to survive much longer than a naked person or one wearing a bathing suit.

These apparently conflicting opinions merely serve to emphasize that patients who are rescued after drowning incidents should not be certified dead until prolonged resuscitation has failed. It may be said again that no patient is dead until he is warm and dead. This particularly applies to infants and small children in whom full neurological recovery has been recorded after up to 45 minutes of asystole.

Miscellaneous problems

Swallowed water Almost every victim of an immersion incident swallows large volumes of fluid before drowning, and this may be important. Hypotonic solutions are rapidly absorbed from the gastrointestinal tract, which may lead to haemodilution and pulmonary oedema. On the other hand, salt water is not well absorbed, and in the author's experience patients who survive sea water immersion often develop severe diarrhoea which may cause dehydration, hypokalaemia and, because of loss of bicarbonate, non-respiratory acidaemia. The fluid loss may be beneficial, the other electrolyte changes may have to be corrected.

Coincidental injuries Many patients who fall or jump into water strike hard objects on the way, and every victim of such an incident should be carefully examined to exclude superficial or internal injuries. On the other hand, coma and accidents due to drugs, alcohol, diabetes, epilepsy and head injury may explain why the patient suffered the immersion incident in the first place. There should be no need to state that every unconscious patient must undergo a full examination to exclude these and other conditions, even if the cause of coma is thought to be obvious. In one series it was reported that 24% of adults involved in immersion incidents had a blood alcohol level greater than 80 mg%.

The treatment of near-drowning

Clean water immersion

Patients who have been immersed in clean water and survive without brain damage usually make a rapid and uncomplicated recovery. On admission to hospital a chest radiograph must be taken and the blood gases measured while the patient is breathing or being ventilated with a known inspired oxygen concentration, either room air if this can be tolerated safely, or 100% oxygen. This allows the Aa gradient to be recorded and demonstrates the extent of the lung damage, and by repeating these observations at intervals which are dictated by the clinical course of the disturbance, its progress can be monitored.

Other baseline data must be obtained. These include a full blood count, serum electrolytes and coagulation screen. Acute renal failure has been recorded on several occasions after immersion incidents, usually attributed to hypoxic tubular damage or to haemolysis. The patient's renal function must be monitored as described in Chapter 2.

Some degree of non-respiratory acidaemia is invariably noted; although this can usually be expected to correct itself in time, if the pH is below 7.25 and the base deficit greater than 10 mmol/l, sodium bicarbonate should be given as described on page 96. However, pulmonary oedema is an ever-present hazard and the volume of sodium bicarbonate infused must be kept to a minimum.

Respiratory care and controlled ventilation The patient should be intubated only if he is unable to guard his airway because of coma, or because he is underventilating or requires controlled ventilation. Although brain damage is the most sinister effect of near-drowning, infection is a close second and water-damaged lungs easily become infected. Endotracheal intubation, controlled ventilation and tracheobronchial toilet increase the hazard of pulmonary infection (and of septicaemia) and if they are necessary, every possible precaution must be taken to minimize these hazards. However, all victims of immersion incidents require graduated oxygen therapy. If the patient has extensive lung damage, as shown radiographically, and is dangerously hypoxic (i.e. PaO_2 less than 7.0 kPa) on 80% oxygen, incremental PEEP should be applied.

The use of diuretics A diuretic such as frusemide should be given although, as mentioned above, patients who have swallowed large quantities of salt water frequently develop severe diarrhoea which may have a similar effect to frusemide.

Secondary drowning was referred to earlier. The treatment of this condition (reactionary pulmonary oedema) also includes the use of diuretics, since although it is not due to circulatory overload or heart failure, diuresis encourages the absorption of water from the lungs by increasing the plasma oncotic pressure.

Recognition and treatment of infection Antibiotics should not be given prophylactically, but sputum specimens must be sent to the microbiological laboratory every day so that bacterial contamination may be recognized and treated quickly and vigorously. With this treatment regimen, most patients are able to leave the ITU within 72 hours of admission, although some may have to stay longer because of other injuries.

If the Aa gradient and radiographic signs do not improve rapidly the possibility of secondary infection or lung damage from unrecognized contamination or aspiration of vomit must be considered. Every unconscious or semiconscious drowning victim is at risk from this latter condition because of the large volume of water swallowed.

Immersion in contaminated water

The prognosis for a patient who has inhaled a large volume of contaminated water is much poorer than that described above—either because of major or minor airway obstruction due to solid material, or because of bacterial or chemical damage to the alveoli. The initial treatment is as described in the last section, although most of the patients will require endotracheal intubation and IPPV from the outset.

Bronchoscopy and tracheobronchial toilet While the patient is being prepared for intubation, bronchoscopy should be performed so that tracheobronchial toilet can be carried out under direct vision and any obvious foreign material removed before the endotracheal tube is passed. After intubation, tracheobronchial lavage should be performed frequently and vigorously until the aspirate is visibly clean. This must be performed aseptically and as atraumatically as possible using up to 25 ml water or normal saline per time.

The prevention or treatment of infection Specimens of sputum and other debris are sent for microbiological examination. Part of the first specimen should be Gram-stained immediately to give some guide to the presence and type of bacterial contamination; this may suggest which antibiotic regimen should be prescribed. Antibacterial treatment cannot hope to eliminate every organism and may simply encourage the emergence of multi-resistant strains of Gram-negative bacteria. However, in the present state of knowledge there is no apparent alternative to this type of blunderbuss therapy. Antibiotics such as polymyxin and gentamicin have also been given by aerosol as adjunctive treatment.

If the contamination is overwhelming, a tracheostomy should be performed early, rather than waiting for seven to ten days as is the normal practice, since tracheobronchial toilet is much more efficient when performed through a tracheostomy.

Cerebral oedema

Any patient who has suffered prolonged hypoxia, with or without ischaemia, is likely to develop acute cerebral oedema manifested by coma or by convulsions together with other signs of raised intracranial pressure. This complication must be recognized immediately and the appropriate treatment applied, which may include the use of diuretics (frusemide or mannitol), hyperventilation, anticonvulsants and continuous intravenous barbiturate or Althesin anaesthesia. The regimen of treatment is described on page 148. Dexamethasone and other corticosteroids are of no value in cerebral oedema due to hypoxia and simply increase the likelihood of overwhelming respiratory tract infection.

References

Airey, I.L., Smith, P.A. & Stoddart, J.C. (1982) Plasma and cerebrospinal fluid barbiturate levels during prolonged continuous thiopentone anaesthesia. *Anaesthesia*, **37**, 328–331.

Calderwood, H.W., Modell, J.H. & Ruiz, B.C. (1975) The ineffectiveness of steroid therapy for treatment of fresh water drowning. *Anesthesiology*, **43**, 642–650.

Clark, R.E., Ordin, L.R. & Rovenstime, E.A. (1954) Body temperature studies in anesthetized man: effect of environmental temperature, humidity and anesthesia system. *Journal of the American Medical Association*, **154**, 311–319.

Conn, A.W. & Modell, J.H. (1980) Current neurological considerations in near-drowning. *Canadian Anaesthetists Society Journal*, **27**, 197–198.

Frates, R.C. (1981) Analysis of predictive factors in the assessment of warm-water near-drowning in children. *American Journal of Diseases of Childhood*, **135**(11), 1006–1008.

Golden, F.St.C. (1980) Problems of immersion. *British Journal of Hospital Medicine*, **4**, 371–383.

Golden, F.St.C. (1980) The management of rescued shipwreck survivors. *Journal of the Royal Naval Medical Service*, **66**, 107–113.

Goldman, A., Exton Smith, A.N., Francis, F. & O'Brien, A. (1977) A pilot study of low body temperature in old people admitted to hospital. *Journal of the Royal College of Physicians, London*, **11**, 291–306.

Hardy, J.D., Gagge, A.P. & Prolwizk, J.A.J. (1970) *Physiological and Behavioural Temperature Regulation*. 191 pp. Springfield, Illinois: Charles C. Thomas.

Holdcroft, A. (1980) *Body Temperature Control*. 130 pp. London: Baillière Tindall.

Laufman, H. (1951) Profound accidental hypothermia. *Journal of the American Medical Association*, **147**, 1201–1212.

Lewis, D.G. & Mackenzie, A. (1972) The effects of mild hypothermia and hyperventilation on acid base balance in major vascular surgery. *British Journal of Anaesthesia*, **44**, 1085–1088.

Maclean, D. & Emslie Smith, D. (1977) *Accidental Hypothermia*. 201 pp. Oxford: Blackwell Scientific.

Modell, J.H., Graves, S.A. & Kuck, E.J. (1980) Near-drowning; correlation of level of consciousness and survival. *Canadian Anaesthetists Society Journal*, **27**, 211–215.

Perkins, M.N., Rothwell, N.J., Stock, M.J. & Stone, T.W. (1981) Activation of brown adipose tissue thermogenesis by the ventromedial hypothalamus. *Nature*, **289**, 401–402.

Rahn, H. (1967) Gas transfer from external environment to cell. In *Development of the Lung* (Ed.) de Reuck, A.V.S. London: Ciba Symposium, Churchill Livingstone.

Reuler, J.B. (1978) Hypothermia; pathophysiology, clinical settings and management. *Annals of Internal Medicine*, **89**, 519–527.

Rivers, J.F., Orr, G. & Lee, H.A. (1970) Drowning: its clinical sequelae and management. *British Medical Journal*, **1**, 157–161.

Russell, W.J. (1974) A review of blood warmers for massive transfusion. *Anaesthesia and Intensive Care*, **2**, 109–130.

Savides, E.P. & Hoffbrand, B.I. (1974) Hypothermia, thrombosis and acute pancreatitis. *British Medical Journal*, **1**, 614.

Siebhe, H., Breivik, H., Rod, T. & Lind, B. (1975) Survival after 40 minutes submersion without cerebral sequelae. *Lancet*, **1**, 1275–1277.

10

Intra-abdominal and Lower Limb Injuries

The anaesthetist who is concerned with the care of the multiply injured patient quickly learns that the external injuries may be only part of the problem, and that occult organ damage and haemorrhage may not become apparent until later when the patient is in the anaesthetic room, the recovery room or the intensive therapy unit.

The recognition and definitive treatment of intra-abdominal injuries is the classic surgical problem, but the anaesthetist must realize the potential for disaster that such injuries may present. In this brief chapter some of these are described.

GUIDELINES TO DIAGNOSIS AND TREATMENT

These may be set out as follows:

History of the injury from the patient or witness

In most cases this can be obtained from the patient, but if he is unconscious or amnesic, a witness to the incident should be found who can describe the sequence of events. The survivors of moving vehicle accidents may present with injuries involving any part of the body, although intracranial, intrathoracic and intra-abdominal injuries present the greatest difficulties. The influence of the seat-belt is referred to later, but the rescue services usually note whether or not it has been worn. Back seat passengers are frequently thrown around the vehicle and may have sustained a wide variety of injuries.

Physical evidence of injury

This may be obvious, with bruising, laceration, penetrating wounds or distortion of the bony configuration. Examples of these include limb deformities, paradoxical ventilation and alteration of the shape of the pelvic brim, but less overt signs include clothing and seat-belt marks. Subcutaneous or intramuscular haematoma are usually obvious, but if the patient is fat or if the haematoma is evenly distributed, its presence may not be noted until discolouration appears days after the injury. The examination of the injured patient must include palpation of the flanks, breasts, buttocks and thighs, areas in which extensive haematomata may be hidden.

It should be pointed out at this stage that closed head injuries never give rise

169

to the classic signs of haemorrhage and an unconscious patient who is shocked must have a source of bleeding which has not been recognized. This is usually inside the abdomen or thoracic cage, although patients may lose a surprisingly large amount of blood from scalp injuries.

Clothing and seat belt marks

At other points in this book the significance of clothing marks has been mentioned. If a patient is found to have a clothing pattern on his chest wall or abdomen—as, for example, the stripes of a shirt or the mesh of an item of underwear—he has probably suffered a major internal injury. Diffuse abrasions caused by traction on clothing are of lesser significance. Some surgeons are prepared to perform an immediate laparotomy if the patient has distinctive clothing marks, although others would be content to observe the patient closely or carry out a pleural tap or peritoneal lavage. In any case, blood must always be cross-matched for this type of patient in anticipation of bleeding which requires resuscitation and surgical treatment.

Seat-belt marks must also be regarded seriously, although patients may be injured by the seat-belt without it marking the skin. The simple lap-strap belt is of little value other than to protect the patient from being thrown out of the car and is often associated with severe facial and head injuries. The combined lap-strap/shoulder-harness seat belt has saved many lives and an even greater number of facial lacerations, but it may also cause significant injuries. These include relatively minor abrasions to the chest and abdominal wall, but a variety of intra-abdominal and some intrathoracic injuries have also been recorded. The commonest involve the spleen, liver and hollow viscera, particularly the duodenojejunal area, although other bowel injuries have been reported. The clavicle may be fractured and the lungs contused; rarely, pericardial tamponade and other intrathoracic injuries may be produced by the seat-belt.

Pain and restricted movements

If a patient complains of abdominal pain which has no obvious external cause, internal injuries must be considered and investigated. Pain which is exacerbated by respiratory movements is suggestive of intraperitoneal bleeding or soiling. The combination of restricted abdominal wall movement and absent bowel sounds has similar implications. The significance of peritonism is obvious although it is often difficult to distinguish from the pain of superficial injuries.

OCCULT BLEEDING

Failure to identify and treat occult bleeding is an important cause of morbidity and death after injury. Although it usually accompanies severe injuries, apparently trivial incidents may be associated with dangerous internal bleeding. The author's first 'death on the table' was a 15-year-old girl who suffered a ruptured spleen when she was thrown over the back of the empty passenger seat when her father swerved to avoid a stray dog. At no time did she complain of pain and it was only when she developed air hunger that the possibility of occult bleeding was considered.

Skeletal injuries

In addition to this type of injury patients with closed pelvic or femoral fractures invariably lose a significant part of their circulating blood volume with no external signs of bleeding. The problem of intrathoracic bleeding is referred to in Chapter 4. Fractures of the ileum and ischium are commonly associated with the loss of 1–2 l blood into the retroperitoneal space. The source of blood loss may not become apparent until bruising appears in the flanks, the buttocks, the perineum and around the inguinal ligament, days after the event. Occasionally major vessels such as the iliac veins are damaged, but open surgical treatment should be avoided because of the risk of infection—although if the inferior vena cava is involved active intervention may be life-saving. The G-suit is often invaluable in this type of injury but it is of no value for the treatment of intraperitoneal bleeding.

A patient with a fractured femoral shaft may lose 0.75–1.5 l blood into the thigh. This may be recognized by comparing its diameter with that of the undamaged leg at the same distance from the anterior superior iliac spine. It is usually stated that the loss of 500 ml blood causes an increase in diameter of 2 cm, although the origin of this statement is lost in medical tradition.

Compound fractures may be obvious and receive the appropriate treatment. However, the attendant must always look carefully for skin puncture wounds over long-bone fractures since these should be regarded as having the same significance.

Patients who have sustained femoral shaft fractures should have radiographs taken of the lumbar spine because avulsion fractures of lumbar transverse processes are sometimes seen. These are usually caused by violent traction on the psoas and iliacus muscles, injuries which are always associated with considerable loss of blood.

Anaesthetic hazards

Whenever the possibility of occult injury exists the anaesthetist must be on the alert. If the patient requires anaesthesia for facio-maxillary, upper or lower limb surgery within a few hours of the injury, central venous pressure monitoring is essential, together with the other routine observations, since a low or falling CVP may be the only sign of bleeding during such manoeuvres and may suggest that further investigations, including a laparotomy, are required.

PENETRATING WOUNDS

From the anaesthetist's standpoint, the most important consideration is the unpredictable nature of penetrating wounds of the abdomen (and/or thorax). He must be prepared for prolonged, extensive and traumatic surgery following what may appear to be a trivial external wound. Extensive haemorrhage, contamination of the peritoneal cavity with intestinal contents, and leakage from the urinary tract may be found. However, the general management of patients suffering from this type of injury is not materially different from that of the inadequately prepared patient who has to undergo any form of emergency abdominal or thoracic surgery.

INVESTIGATION OF INTRA-ABDOMINAL INJURIES

The clinical signs are often so conclusive that no further investigation is required and the patient may be taken straight to the operating room. In other cases plain abdominal, semi-erect and lateral decubitus radiographs may reveal the presence of gas under the diaphragm, an abnormal number of fluid levels, or that one or other diaphragm is displaced, leading to suspicion of the presence of fluid, usually blood, beneath it. Fractures of lower ribs on either side may cause injury to the spleen or liver and explain the origin of occult bleeding. Very occasionally, fractured ribs may be associated with damage to the stomach or other hollow viscera.

It was stated in Chapter 4 that if a patient with chest injuries requires sedation and controlled ventilation, the attendant must be sure that he has no coincidental intra-abdominal injuries. A negative laparotomy is not a disaster, but two alternative methods of investigation exist, namely, quadrantic aspiration and peritoneal lavage.

Quadrantic aspiration and peritoneal lavage

Quadrantic aspiration is performed by inserting a size 16 intravenous cannula into the peritoneal cavity in each flank, the epigastrium and the suprapubic region, while aspirating with a 20 ml syringe. Occasionally, irrefutable evidence of intra-abdominal bleeding is obtained, but both false-positive and false-negative results are common and it is quite easy to perforate distended bowel.

Peritoneal lavage is a much better technique. Several methods are available, but the simplest is to insert a peritoneal dialysis catheter by the standard technique 2–3 cm below the umbilicus and irrigate 100 ml aliquots of saline through it. If the effluent is consistently blood-stained or soiled with intestinal contents, the patient requires a laparotomy.

At various stages in this book, traumatic pancreatic damage is mentioned and this should always be suspected as a cause of major systemic disturbance. However, both the serum amylase and the peritoneal fluid amylase may be elevated if the patient has a contused pancreas, without causing other symptoms.

As many as 22% of patients who have suffered pelvic fractures also have intra-peritoneal injuries in addition to the haematoma. If peritoneal lavage is performed via the usual sub-umbilical site it may give false-positive information since pelvic haematomas frequently extend up the anterior abdominal wall. This possibility must always be borne in mind.

Whichever method of peritoneal lavage is performed, the patient's bladder must be known to be empty beforehand, so as to avoid the risk of perforation with the needle or peritoneal dialysis catheter.

The 'mini-laparotomy'

At present there is a vogue for performing the 'mini-laparotomy' through a 5 cm para-umbilical incision. Although this may permit obvious signs of intra-abdominal injury to be recognized it cannot guarantee to demonstrate subphrenic, pelvic or retroperitoneal injury; most experienced anaesthetists and surgeons know that if the patient can tolerate a mini-laparotomy he can equally well tolerate a formal exploratory procedure, which provides much more reliable information.

GENITOURINARY TRACT INJURIES

Responsibility for the definitive treatment of genitourinary tract (GU) injuries rests with the relevant surgical specialist. However, because the anaesthetist is usually involved at an early stage in the resuscitation of the trauma victim and may occasionally be the most senior person present, he should be aware of the problems and pitfalls which GU injuries present. In addition, the patient may be admitted to the ITU before suspicion of GU injury is aroused.

In most cases the problem is that of occult bleeding, and the treatment proceeds upon the general lines already discussed. The G-suit may be life-saving for the patient with severe retroperitoneal bleeding from pelvic and lumbar vertebral fractures. However, in others, damage to the kidneys, ureters, bladder and urethra may create major difficulties.

Urethral catheterization

The most immediate problem is concerned with the attendant's desire to monitor the urine output. If the patient could possibly have sustained injuries to the pubis or perineum, a urinary catheter should not be passed until a GU surgeon has been asked his opinion, since it may aggravate any injury to the urethra or bladder neck. If such an opinion cannot be obtained, the medical attendant must make a series of observations and investigations before doing anything which may harm the patient. The following points must be considered.

1 Has the patient had time to need to pass urine since the accident? No attempt should be made to pass a catheter until at least two hours after the accident.

2 Has the patient passed any urine since the accident? If so, was it blood-stained or was micturition painful or difficult? His clothing must be examined, since many patients pass urine involuntarily after accidents.

3 Is there any blood in the patient's underclothing or at the tip of the urethra? This suggests the presence of urethral injury.

4 Does the patient have signs suggestive of a full bladder?

5 Are there any signs of extravasation of urine in the lower abdominal wall, the perineum or external genitalia?

Radiological investigation of urinary tract injuries

If damage to the urethra or bladder neck is suspected, 15 ml of a water-soluble radiographic contrast medium such as Conray 40 may be gently instilled through a catheter passed not more than 2 cm into the urethra. This should flow into the bladder, but a radiograph may show extravasation or obstruction. In either case no attempt to catheterize the patient should be made until a GU surgeon has been contacted. If the bladder is obviously distended because of bladder neck obstruction, a suprapubic cystotomy will probably need to be performed. This may be performed in the operating room, although a selection of prepacked kits is available so that it can safely be performed under local anaesthesia in the patient's bed.

If, as so often happens, the patient has already been catheterized before admission to the ITU but there is a question of injury to the lower genitourinary tract, a cystogram should be performed through the catheter. This will show evidence of leakage from the bladder or the urethra. If this is trivial and the bladder will accept 400–500 ml urine, there is no need for surgical treatment, although many GU surgeons recommend that prophylactic antibiotics should be given.

If the patient has haematuria but is producing an adequate volume of urine, an intravenous urogram (IVU) should be performed. This can be done quite satisfactorily in the ITU and films should be taken at ten-minute and fifteen-minute intervals after injection of the contrast medium. The renal outline, the ureters and the bladder should all be visible. If only one kidney is identifiable it may be advisable to perform a renal angiogram. The position of the ureter may be displaced because of retroperitoneal haematoma.

Very occasionally both ureters are obstructed by a pelvic haematoma and consequently the patient is anuric. This condition should be diagnosed very quickly, but it may not be considered until the patient has been anuric for some hours. Provided it is recognized promptly no harm should result; an intravenous urogram will show both kidneys to be excreting the dye, together with the dilatation of both ureters. This is an indication for surgical intervention irrespective of the patient's other injuries.

The IVU may show distortion of one or both renal pelves or demonstrate that part of one kidney is not outlined by the nephrogram. Occasionally the dye may be noticed to extravasate from some part of the GU tract. All of these abnormal findings must be regarded as urgent indications for obtaining expert advice.

References

Bergqvist, D., Hedelin, H. & Lindblad, B. (1980) Blunt renal trauma. *Scandinavian Journal of Urology and Nephrology*, **14,** 177–181.

Flint, L.M., Brown, A., Richardson, J.D. & Polk, H.C. (1979) Definitive control of bleeding from severe pelvic fractures. *Annals of Surgery*, **189,** 709–712.

Jergens, M.E. (1977) Peritoneal lavage. *American Journal of Surgery*, **133,** 365–368.

Krausz, M.M., Mauny, J., Utsunomiyn, T. & Hechtman, H.B. (1981) Peritoneal lavage in blunt abdominal trauma. *Surgery, Gynecology and Obstetrics*, **152,** 327–330.

London, P.S. (1967) *A Practical Guide to the Care of the Injured.* 777 pp. Edinburgh and London: Churchill Livingstone.

Pedersey, S. & Jansen, V. (1979) Intestinal lesions caused by incorrectly placed seat belts. *Acta Chirurgica Scandinavica*, **145**, 15–20.

Walt, A.J. (1980) Major problems in blunt and penetrating abdominal trauma. *Canadian Journal of Surgery*, **23**, 343–347.

11

Transporting the Injured Patient

Transporting patients who have suffered severe physical injury (or who are otherwise incapacitated) is often considered to present insuperable problems; many patients who would have benefited from specialized attention, but who were believed to be too ill to move, have died because of this fear. There is no doubt that certain difficulties do exist, but experience has shown that provided that the patient is properly prepared for the journey and accompanied by skilled personnel, which in most cases should include an anaesthetist, the journey itself should pass without incident. On general principles it is better to avoid excessive movement and unnecessary handling, and the best modern ambulance or other form of transport is not entirely free from noise, roll and vibration, but these are surprisingly innocuous for even the most seriously ill patient. In the United Kingdom, journeys of this kind should rarely exceed two hours' duration.

On the Continent, and with increasing frequency in the United Kingdom, helicopters and fixed wing aircraft are used to transport the critically ill or dependent patient over long distances. It is usually stated that helicopter flights should not exceed 75 miles radius but much longer distances have been covered in emergencies. In Australia, patients are frequently moved thousands of miles by air without coming to any harm. The problems which are presented by these two forms of transport are not materially different from those which are created by standard methods, although helicopters are notoriously noisy and vibration may create practical difficulties.

Some of the difficulties which surround the transport of large numbers of casualties were outlined in Chapter 1. In this circumstance only first aid is possible, based upon the triad of guaranteeing the patency of the airway, controlling or assisting breathing and supporting the circulation. However, when only one patient has to be moved the journey should be an unhurried, properly planned, and carefully executed manoeuvre.

PRE-TRANSFER PREPARATION AND TREATMENT

In the last 12 years more than 250 very sick patients (not all the victims of trauma) have been transferred to the author's ITU from other hospitals over distances ranging from three to 66 miles, without one death in transit and without any evidence of major physical disturbance. The patient's condition is first discussed by telephone and in most cases an immediate decision can be made that he needs to be transferred. The responsibility for making the transport arrangements is taken by the transferring hospital. No specialized facilities exist in this region but the ambulance services have a wide experience of this type of work. Before the patient is moved the investigations and treatment which are outlined later in this section are performed. In approximately 30% of cases the author or a colleague visits the referring hospital to ensure that the patient both needs and can benefit from the move. This visit is always worthwhile because it often reveals that the patient is receiving all the treatment he needs or, alternatively, that no further treatment can help him.

Pre-transfer assessment

Conditions which may be aggravated by movement include skull fractures, cervical and lumbar spine injuries or other major injuries which may cause occult bleeding or sudden deterioration in the patient's level of consciousness. Therefore, before the patient is moved, these must be identified and treated. However, there is no doubt that the most dangerous problems are asphyxia and respiratory failure, caused either by the underlying condition or its treatment, and these events must be prevented or catered for.

A full pre-transfer clinical examination must be performed to allow an estimate to be made of the severity of the obvious injuries and of the likelihood of hitherto unrecognized complications occurring. Although the patient's renal and hepatic function may also be impaired and present long-term problems, all that is usually necessary before the patient is moved is an assessment of the state of his cardiocirculatory, respiratory and central nervous systems.

Most of the data required can be obtained from the referring hospital's pulse, blood pressure and fluid balance charts. The patient's urine output per hour must be known. If these show instability or deterioration in any of the vital parameters, it may be necessary either to delay transfer until further treatment has been administered, or, in the case of neurological problems, either abandon or accelerate it. Any evidence which suggests that the patient's level of consciousness is deteriorating or that focal neurological signs are emerging must be acted upon.

The observed rate of blood loss and its replacement must be noted to allow an estimate to be made of the volume of blood or other transfusion fluids which may be needed during the projected journey. All of the record charts must be provided so that on arrival at the receiving hospital the observations can be continued. As described later, essential observations must be recorded during transit. A list should be made of all of the investigations which have been undertaken before the patient is moved and the transfer team should be provided with some vital data. These include:

1 Full blood count
2 Blood gas analysis figures
3 Urea and electrolyte results
4 Blood group

The appropriate radiographs should be available. These *must* include a chest radiograph taken within one hour of the commencement of the journey; the tip of the endotracheal tube must be visible on the erect radiograph so that endobronchial intubation can be excluded.

Pre-transfer treatment

In transit only minimal resuscitation and monitoring are possible unless the facilities are of an ultrasophisticated nature. Therefore, all essential treatment must be established before the journey begins. This may include:

1   Fixation or splinting of major fractures
2   Establishment of essential intravenous lines
3   The provision of all of the intravenous fluids which may be required during the journey, including blood, PPF and electrolyte solutions
4   Endotracheal intubation
5   The insertion of chest drains and urinary catheters

Airway care

As nearly as possible all artificial airways must be guaranteed free from kinking, displacement or disconnection since unquestionably these are the greatest hazards of the journey. It is safer to transport a patient with an endotracheal (nasotracheal) tube in place than one who has very recently acquired a tracheostomy. If it is planned to perform a tracheostomy, this should be deferred until the patient reaches his destination. Fresh tracheostomy wounds not infrequently bleed, particularly if the patient has to be moved. If a tracheostomy is less than two days old and the tube becomes displaced, it may be quite difficult to re-insert, particularly in a moving vehicle. If the accident occurs the attendant should follow the recommendations made on page 69, and first pass an orotracheal tube to achieve control of the airway. In most cases no attempt should be made to re-insert the tracheostomy tube until the vehicle has stopped or, preferably, until the receiving hospital is reached.

For reasons which have already been stated (page 67), nasotracheal plastic tubes are usually preferred to orotracheal, rubber or reinforced tubes. The tube must be cut to the right length so that only the minimum length protrudes from the nostril or mouth. Long tubes tend to kink or advance down the right main bronchus. Nylon reinforced tubes have some apparent advantages, but they may spring out of the trachea if the head and neck are moved abruptly and are then difficult to re-insert, with or without an introducer, in a moving vehicle. All connectors must be checked before the journey begins; these include ventilator hoses, catheter mounts and tube connectors. No apology is offered for making such apparently obvious recommendations since disconnection, or the inability to join tubes together, are common causes of difficulty or disaster when patients have to be moved.

Chest drainage

If the patient has a chest drain in place, it is usually safer and more convenient to connect this to a Heimlich-type dry valve rather than to the standard underwater drain, unless blood or other fluid is draining freely.

If the patient has sustained chest wall injuries but as yet has no evidence of a pneumothorax and he is receiving controlled ventilation, serious consideration must be given to the desirability of inserting a drain into one or both sides of the chest before he is placed in the ambulance. In an ambulance the diagnosis of pneumothorax may be virtually impossible, and if the drains are inserted aseptically before the journey begins, and with care, no harm should result.

SEDATION AND/OR ANAESTHESIA FOR THE PATIENT IN TRANSIT

If the patient is conscious, breathing spontaneously and in pain the choice and dose of analgesic drug is a matter for personal preference. Whichever agent is used its effects must be continuously monitored and the attendant should be prepared to deal with any undesirable complication in transit.

Entonox may be effective, although for long journeys its use creates the additional difficulties of bulk and supply and occasionally the patient using it may become restless and confused. However, he should at least be well oxygenated.

Incremental, low dose, intravenous morphine is almost certainly the safest and most effective substance to use. In any case the effects of the selected agent should be assessed before the journey begins, both because all analgesics are better given in anticipation of pain than after it has begun, and to estimate the drug's desirable and undesirable effects.

If the patient is intubated and receiving controlled ventilation the choice is simplified. Any analgesic in an adequate dose may be given and it should be possible to make the patient completely pain-free and amnesic for the journey. If he requires pancuronium or other muscle relaxant the attendant must be absolutely certain that he is neither in pain nor emotionally distressed when the relaxant is given. In this situation ketamine may be the agent of choice since its dose/response relationship is very predictable and its cardiovascular side-effects minimal. Benzodiazepines such as diazepam should be used only if the patient is not in pain since they have no analgesic properties and are unpredictable sedatives with even more unpredictable cardiorespiratory side-effects.

MONITORING AND TREATMENT IN TRANSIT

Continuous observation and record-keeping present major problems. These are normally regarded as being essential requirements in any traumatized patient, but they are difficult to satisfy in a moving vehicle. Therefore a skilled observer who is able to make clinical judgements using only his eyes and hands must accompany the patient. Neither the stethoscope nor standard sphygmomanometer can be used in an ambulance or helicopter. Intravascular monitoring is likewise difficult because of vibration and gross movements. Very sophisticated transport systems which rely upon large aircraft equipped with every conceivable monitoring and therapeutic device have been made available for crowned heads and presidents.

Equipping the ambulance

Monitoring

Battery-powered intravascular pressure monitoring systems have been constructed but are not widely used. However, there are many battery-powered ECG–defibrillator combinations available which are relatively unaffected by physical movement or electrical interference. If the patient is receiving oxygen therapy or IPPV his inspired oxygen concentration can be monitored with a portable polarographic electrode which also serves as a disconnection or oxygen failure alarm. This is an appropriate point to state that before the patient is moved, the attendant must be absolutely certain that all of the services which he requires, including oxygen, are guaranteed for the anticipated duration of the journey. A generous allowance must be made for delays caused by traffic hold-ups and mechanical breakdown.

Intravenous therapy

The administration of intravenous therapy should not rely upon gravity; all infusions should be pressurized and drugs such as narcotics, sedatives or relaxants should be given continuously by battery-operated syringe pumps. The intravenous line(s) should be established and secured before the patient leaves his home base and infusion sites must not be obscured by dressings.

Suction

A reliable source of suction is absolutely essential so that oropharyngeal and tracheobronchial toilet can be performed. Oxygen-powered venturi-type suction is the most efficient, although it uses large quantities of oxygen which may create supply problems on long journeys. Foot-operated suction units are very effective when stationary but are difficult to use reliably in a moving vehicle. Disposable vacuum suckers are of little use since they quickly become exhausted.

Basic equipment

Wherever possible, all of the treatment which is necessary should be established before the ambulance leaves its home base. However, instruments and pre-packed dressings should be carried in the ambulance or other transport so that wounds can be re-dressed if necessary. Rolls of 2″ elastoplast, domette bandages and dressing scissors are most often needed. If the patient has a tracheostomy the kit must include tracheal dilators. If he has a chest drain in situ, a replacement should be provided in case it should become displaced; a chest drainage kit should be provided whenever a patient with chest injuries is being moved, although the problems which surround the recognition of pneumothorax have already been referred to.

Replacements for intravenous cannulae and infusion sets should also be carried. It is unlikely that a patient could fill a urine bag during the average journey undertaken within the United Kingdom, but all urine passed must be retained for analysis.

Controlled ventilation in transit

For journeys of less than 30 minutes' duration there is little doubt that
hand-ventilation with oxygen-enriched air from a device such as the Ambu
bag is the simplest and safest. However, if the medical attendant expects to
have other things to do during the journey, or if this is prolonged, a
mechanical ventilator should be used. Standard operating room machines can
be used and, with proper organization and the availability of nitrous oxide
and oxygen cylinders, patients can be anaesthetized throughout the journey.
Both pressure-cycled and minute volume divider type ventilators have been
used successfully.

Many simple systems are available which are designed to be economical in
gas consumption and still be able to provide a variety of flow, pressure and
oxygen delivery patterns. These include the 'Blease', 'Oxylog' and 'Pneupac'
ranges which may be powered by oxygen, with air mix, or with entonox, and
journeys of up to three hours' duration are possible without having to change
cylinders. The choice depends upon personal preference and cost.

If transporting patients between hospitals is expected to be a frequent and
regular requirement, other provisions may be made. One system comprises a
self-contained patient trolley which carries a ventilator, pressurized gases, a
basic anaesthetic machine and monitoring devices which can be lifted
hydraulically into a modified ambulance. With the cooperation of the
ambulance services and the Treasury, almost any degree of sophistication is
attainable although it is probably unnecessary.

AMBULANCE DESIGN

Size, roominess, heating, lighting and suspension must be of the highest order
obtainable. Systems which are converted from estate cars have been devised
by enthusiasts but they suffer from the major drawback that the medical
attendant cannot perform therapeutic manoeuvres in transit because of lack
of space. Hopefully, when it is recognized that regional services for the
treatment of trauma victims are both more efficient and more economic,
ambulance design will be more specialized. The standard high, wide
wheel-based vehicle provides a satisfactory basis upon which modifications
can be made, although the standard suspension leaves much to be desired.

Basic ambulance requirements

The basic requirements are:
1 Freedom from mechanical breakdown
2 Spaciousness
3 Good suspension
4 Sound insulation
5 Good interior lighting and heating

Some special facilities may be necessary. These include:
1 An adjustable operating light

2   Electrical power points
3   Storage racks for oxygen and nitrous oxide cylinders
4   Interference-free radio communication
5   A reliable source of suction
6   Drug and equipment cabinets

The need for electrical outlets is rapidly being superseded by the increasing availability of battery-operated monitoring equipment. The major anxiety during most journeys is the exhaustion of gas cylinders, and the consumption of gases per hour must be calculated before the journey begins and an adequate replacement supply carried.

Communications

During the journey, communication between the accompanying doctor and driver and between the ambulance, its home station and destination must be as interference-free as possible. This is particularly important in case of mechanical breakdown, but it may be necessary to ask the driver to stop if an emergency occurs inside the ambulance, such as endotracheal tube displacement or the appearance of signs of a tension pneumothorax. It may be necessary to inform the receiving hospital of some new development so that treatment may be instituted as soon as the patient arrives. Similarly, if the patient dies in transit the reception team can be saved an unnecessary wait.

The drug and equipment cabinet design and its contents are a matter for personal choice, but access, display and labelling should be given priority. A minimum of essential equipment should be carried in containers which are always held ready for patient transport; specialized drugs and equipment can be added to the basic contents according to the anticipated needs of the patient. The essentials include:

1   Airways (including nasopharyngeal tubes)
2   Cuffed endotracheal tubes already prepared with angle mounts
3   Endotracheal tube stilette
4   Laryngoscope (long and paediatric blades)
5   Ambu bag and face-masks
6   Magill forceps
7   Mouth gag
8   Syringes, needles
9   Intravenous cannulae and catheters
10 Infusion sets
11 Basic infusion fluids—plasma protein fraction, gelatine solution, Dextran 70, sodium bicarbonate 8.4%, Hartmann's solution, dextrose 5% in water
12 Complete chest drain pack and suture pack
13 Large basic pack (gauze, swabs, etc.)
14 Essential instruments—surgical scissors, artery clips, tourniquet, dressing scissors
15 Domette bandages, 2″ Elastoplast, 4″ crepe bandages

The drug selection should include:
1   Analgesics—phenoperidine, morphine, ketamine;

2 Sedatives—diazepam emulsion or midazolam;
3 Vasoactive substances—atropine, adrenaline, dopamine, isoprenaline, calcium chloride, ouabaine;
4 Antidysrhythmics—lignocaine infusion, disopyramide, atenolol;
5 Muscle relaxants—pancuronium, suxamethonium;
6 Miscellaneous substances—dextrose 50%, insulin, naloxone.

Some of these substances have a finite life and the contents of the pack must be checked regularly. Narcotics cannot be stored inside vehicles which may at times be used by the general public, and unless the vehicle is kept for the exclusive use of the emergency team, the drugs and equipment cabinets should be stored inside the hospital. The ITU or casualty department is the logical place for this, and the checking and replenishing of the contents can then be the responsibility of the appropriate nursing staff.

A G-suit (or MAST suit) and space blanket are commonly required in addition to the equipment described above. These and other special items are added when needed.

References

Adams, A.P. & Henville, J.D. (1977) A new generation of anaesthetic ventilators. *Anaesthesia*, **32**, 34–40.

Aitkenhead, A.R., Willis, M.I. & Barnes, W.H. (1980) An economical mobile intensive care unit. *British Medical Journal*, **1**, 1219–1221.

Gray, A.J.G. (1981) Portable lung ventilators. *British Journal of Hospital Medicine*, **2**, 173–178.

Harber, T. & Lucas, B.G.B. (1980) An evaluation of some mechanical resuscitators for use in the ambulance service. *Annals of the Royal College of Surgeons*, **62**, 290–293.

Hothensall, A.P., Waddell, G., Smith, H.C. et al (1977) Mobile intensive care; II. secondary transport. In *Recent Advances in Intensive Therapy*. (Ed.) Ledingham, I.McA. Chapter 18. Edinburgh and London: Churchill Livingstone.

Lambrew, C.T. (1977) Mobile intensive care; I. primary transport. In *Recent Advances in Intensive Therapy*. (Ed.) Ledingham, I.McA. Chapter 17. Edinburgh and London: Churchill Livingstone.

Marsh, R.H.K. & Ledingham, I.McA. (1981) Equipment for mobile intensive care. *British Journal of Hospital Medicine*, **4**, 377–385.

Index

Illustrations are indicated by *italics*.

184